CUTANEOUS
TOXICITY

Academic Press Rapid Manuscript Reproduction

Proceedings of the Third Conference on Cutaneous Toxicity,
Washington, D.C., May 16–18, 1976, Sponsored by the American
Medical Association and the Society of Toxicology

CUTANEOUS TOXICITY

edited by

Victor A. Drill, M.D., Ph.D.
Paul Lazar, M.D.

1977

Academic Press Inc.   NEW YORK   SAN FRANCISCO   LONDON
A Subsidiary of Harcourt Brace Jovanovich, Publishers

ACADEMIC PRESS, INC.
111 Fifth Avenue, New York, New York 10003

United Kingdom Edition published by
ACADEMIC PRESS, INC. (LONDON) LTD.
24/28 Oval Road, London NW1

Library of Congress Cataloging in Publication Data

Conference on Cutaneous Toxicity, 3d, Washington,
    D. C., 1976.
    Cutaneous toxicity.

    Bibliography: p.
    Includes index.
    1.   Toxicology, Experimental–Congresses.
2.   Dermatology, Experimental–Congresses.   3.   Skin
absorption–Congresses.   I.   Drill, Victor
Alexander,   Date   II.   Lazar, Paul.   III.   Ameri-
can Medical Association.   IV.   Society of Toxicology.
V.   Title.
RA1199.C65   1976   616.5   76-30283
ISBN 0–12–222050–1

CONTENTS

PARTICIPANTS

DONALD J. BIRMINGHAM, Department of Dermatology and Syphilology, Wayne State University School of Medicine, Detroit, Michigan 48201

JOSEPH F. BORZELLECA, Department of Pharmacology, Medical College of Virginia, Virginia Commonwealth University, Richmond, Virginia 23298

MARY K. BRUCH, Division of Anti-Infective Drug Products, Bureau of Drugs, Food and Drug Administration, Rockville, Maryland 20852

DAVID J. BRUSICK, Department of Genetics, Litton Bionetics, Inc., Kensington, Maryland 20795

EDWIN V. BUEHLER, Miami Valley Laboratories, The Procter & Gamble Company, Cincinnati, Ohio 45247

CLYDE M. BURNETT, Clairol Research Laboratory, Stamford, Connecticut 06902

S. K. CHANDRASEKARAN, ALZA Research, Palo Alto, California 94304

JOHN F. CORBETT, Clairol Research Laboratory, Stamford, Connecticut 06902

VICTOR A. DRILL, Department of Pharmacology, University of Illinois College of Medicine, Chicago, Illinois 60680

ROBERT B. DROTMAN, Miami Valley Laboratories, The Procter & Gamble Company, Cincinnati, Ohio 45247

THOMAS F. EAGLETON, United States Senate, Washington, D.C. 20510

SEYMOUR L. FRIESS, Environmental Biosciences Department, U.S. Naval Medical Research Institute, Bethesda, Maryland 20014

PETER J. FROSCH, Department of Dermatology, University of Pennsylvania School of Medicine, Philadelphia, Pennsylvania 19104

LOUISA GEHLMANN, Department of Dermatology, Rush-Presbyterian-St. Luke's Medical Center, Rush University, Chicago, Illinois 60612

ROBERT P. GIOVACCHINI, Gillette Medical Evaluation Laboratories, Rockville, Maryland 20850

JOHN F. GRIFFITH, Ivorydale Technical Center, The Procter & Gamble Company, Cincinnati, Ohio 45217

DOROTHY B. HOOD, Haskell Laboratory for Toxicology and Industrial Medicine, E. I. duPont & Company, Newark, Delaware 19711

JOSEPH B. JEROME, Department of Drugs, American Medical Association, Chicago, Illinois 60610

NAOMI M. KANOF, Department of Dermatology, Georgetown University School of Medicine, Washington, D.C. 20036

ALBERT M. KLIGMAN, Department of Dermatology, University of Pennsylvania School of Medicine, Philadelphia, Pennsylvania 19104

PAUL LAZAR, Department of Dermatology, Northwestern University Medical School, Chicago, Illinois 60611

HOWARD I. MAIBACH, Department of Dermatology, University of California Medical School in San Francisco, San Francisco, California 94122

FREDERICK D. MALKINSON, Department of Dermatology, Rush-Presbyterian–St. Luke's Medical Center, Rush University, Chicago, Illinois 60612

GEORGE F. MALLISON, Bacterial Diseases Division, Bureau of Epidemiology, Center for Disease Control, U.S. Public Health Service, H.E.W., Atlanta, Georgia 30333

FRANCIS N. MARZULLI, Toxicology Division, Food & Drug Administration, Washington, D.C. 20036

ALBERT E. MUNSON, Department of Pharmacology, Medical College of Virginia, Virginia Commonwealth University, Richmond, Virginia 23298

ADOLPH ROSTENBERG, JR., Department of Dermatology, University of Illinois College of Medicine, Chicago, Illinois 60680

JANE E. SHAW, ALZA Research, Palo Alto, California 94304

JEROME L. SHUPACK, Department of Dermatology, New York University School of Medicine, New York, New York 10016

ALLEN C. STEERE, JR., Infectious Disease and Rheumatology Department, Yale-New Haven Hospital, New Haven, Connecticut 06510

RONALD C. WESTER, Research Division, Searle Laboratories, Skokie, Illinois 60076

FOREWORD

This volume includes papers presented at the Third Conference on Cutaneous Toxicity co-sponsored by the American Medical Association and the Society of Toxicology and held May 16–18, 1976, in Washington, D.C. As with the published proceedings of the earlier conferences, these papers highlight recent progress, current problems, and future needs in the many specialized activities whose sum total is included in the phrase cutaneous toxicity. Dr. Drill's Introduction provides a succinct review of these scientific considerations as they have developed over the years.

This series of conferences and conference proceedings is a tribute to the co-sponsoring organizations who have provided the organizational resources in terms of personnel and facilities to make them possible.

With respect to the Third Conference, two men bore the primary responsibility from initial program planning to the completion of the editorial tasks for these proceedings. They are Victor A. Drill, M.D., for the Society, and Paul Lazar, M.D., for the AMA; they have carried out their duties in a cooperative spirit with dedication and distinction. The co-chairmen worked under the supervision and benign guidance of Seymour L. Friess, Ph.D., President of the Society, and Asher J. Finkel, M.D., Senior Vice-President for Scientific Activities of the AMA.

The co-sponsors are grateful to the Society of Cosmetic Chemists, which, through a number of its chapters, helped bring pre-Conference publicity to the attention of its members. The professional and trade publications serving physicians, toxicologists, pharmacologists, as well as drug and cosmetic industry scientists provided welcome publicity and informative reports.

The panel of speakers and moderators, reflecting their own work and that of their colleagues, was of course the heart of the Conference.

All the above, whose labors are not readily measured, will feel gratified if their contributions will serve as topics for discussion, potential well-springs for ideas for further research, or sparks for the intellectual curiosity of their listening and reading audiences.

It has once again, as for both earlier conferences, been my pleasant experience to assist in the coordination of some of the supportive staff activities.

Joseph B. Jerome, Ph.D.
Senior Scientist, AMA

Cutaneous Toxicity: Introduction

Victor A. Drill

Department of Pharmacology
University of Illinois School of Medicine
Chicago, Illinois

This is the Third Conference on Cutaneous Toxicity sponsored by the Department of Drugs of the American Medical Association and the Society of Toxicology. The first two conferences in this series were held in 1964 and 1968, and it is timely that we meet again to review some of the problems, the developments, and the advances in knowledge that have been made in the last eight years. The conference thus brings together investigators from a variety of disciplines and provides an opportunity to discuss various aspects of cutaneous toxicity in relation to the safety of drugs and chemicals for man.

Cutaneous reactions may occur in response to a variety of societal situations. Certainly, with regard to drugs, the skin is more commonly affected by an adverse drug reaction than any other organ system. Reactions may also occur following exposure to chemicals encountered in chemical industry, manufacturing processes of various types, from cosmetics and related materials applied to the skin, and from gaseous and solid substances in the air. Other factors that can influence the occurrence of a reaction, and which should not be forgotten, include mechanical irritation, sunlight, and ambient temperature and humidity. It is just over 30 years ago that Draize *et al.* (1) reported their assay for the evaluation of irritation potential in the rabbit. It may be estimated that about 10 to 15 years were required before we began to understand the correlation between animal and human irritation tests and thereby to evaluate the predictability of the Draize procedure for man, and papers on this relationship are still appearing in the literature. During this time span both the experimental and clinical test procedures were modified a number of times by various investigators. I mention these factors because of the common tendency to adopt and give weight to new testing procedures before adequately assessing the test in question; study and evaluation take time and there is no substitute for obtaining the basic knowledge and data required to validate new methodology.

It is of interest to look back 30 years and see some of the changes that have occurred relative to our understanding of cutaneous reactions. In teaching pharmacology in the 1940s we were concerned very simply with discussion of some of the regimens, largely empirical in nature, which were available for the treatment of skin diseases, and a listing of cutaneous reactions reported to occur from drugs and chemicals. We presented little if any basic data regarding the skin and perhaps tended to consider the skin mainly as a relatively inert barrier. All of this has now changed. Today we emphasize the fact that skin is a metabolically active tissue utilizing, for example, glucose and responding to insulin, and synthesizing, among other things, lipids and sterols. An increasing amount of definitive data has also become available on cutaneous absorption and the metabolic transformations which take place in the skin. The prostaglandins, which have been isolated from a variety of body organs, appear to be metabolic regulators required for certain normal biological functions, and some pathological situations are associated with an excess production of prostaglandins. Several prostaglandins have been recognized as mediators of the inflammatory response, and other reports demonstrate that aspirin can inhibit prostaglandin synthesis, which may explain the anti-inflammatory action of aspirin. Significantly, it has now been reported that prostaglandin E_2 is synthesized by skin (2). Further knowledge of the function of prostaglandins in skin may add to our understanding of the process of irritation and other manifestations of cutaneous toxicity. When the Fourth Conference on Cutaneous Toxicity is convened we can confidently expect to have added further to our knowledge of cutaneous toxicity.

REFERENCES

1. Draize, J. H., Woodward, G., and Calvery, H. O. (1944).
    Methods for the study of irritation and toxicity of substances applied topically to skin and mucous membranes.

J. Pharmacol. Exp., Ther. 82:377.

2. Ziboh, V. A., and Hsia, S. L. (1971). Prostaglandin E :
    Biosynthesis and effects on glucose and lipid metabolism.
    Arch. Biochem. Biophys. 146:100

What Is a Reaction:
Factors in the Interpretation
and Reporting of Cosmetic Data

Paul Lazar

Department of Dermatology
Northwestern University Medical School
Chicago, Illinois

Do you remember an old Indo-Persian story about "The Blind Men and the Elephant"? For those who have never read it or have forgotten, the tale is about six blind men who examined an elephant. Each felt a different part of the animal and described what he felt. The ear was thought to be a fan, the leg a tree trunk, the side a wall, the tusk a spear, the trunk a rope, and the tail a snake. The blind men argued about the description of the elephant. Finally, the wise Rajah explained, "You must put all the parts together to find out what an elephant is like." For this occasion, to find the whole truth about cosmetic reactions, we must put all the parts together.

Who are the blind of this talk? They are the physicians and scientists, industry representatives, those in government, consumers, statisticians, and news reporters.

The marrow of this situation has as its elements prejudice, misinformation, poor technique, inability to comprehend the problem, sales promotion, and the desire for power. To fix the word "reaction," the unabridged edition of the *Random House Dictionary of the English Language* defines a reaction as a response to some influence or event. However, the events and influences are many, and the definition of a reaction may vary considerably, depending upon the training, knowledge, and point of view of the interpreter. Let us review, then, some of the problems and opinions regarding

5

cosmetic reactions as viewed by the physician, the government, the consumer, the press, and the statistician.

THE PHYSICIAN-SCIENTIST

   In general, the spectrum of physicians' knowledge, interest, and training as related to cutaneous reactions to
cosmetics is quite broad. However, few physicians are well
trained or experienced in contact allergy, let alone have the
interest in or take the time to do patch testing. Some physicians don't like to be labeled as cosmeticians or want to
be bothered with this area of medicine. The vast majority
of purported reactions to cosmetics and topically applied
chemicals are supported only by clinical appearance and history, and only infrequently are good patch testing techniques
applied. Practically all the medical expertise exists within
small groups in the specialties of dermatology, allergy, and
occupational medicine. This unfortunate situation results
from lack of interest on the physician's part, inadequate
training, inadequate time available to perform such investigations properly and frequently, and the patient's unwilling-
ness to spend the time or money needed for such work. Industrial secrecy, fear of litigation, and poor governmental
efforts in the area also retard advancement.
   The allergic skin reaction to chemicals is much less
common than the irritant reaction. This was always emphasized strongly by one of my teachers, the late Dr. Louis
Schwartz. Despite this, allergic contact dermatitis has been
studied more extensively than irritant reactions, in part because irritation is a more difficult concept to evaluate. In
addition, there is a certain romance in roaming through the
beautiful gardens of common antigens, cross-reactivity,
photoallergic responses, and the allergic contact phenomenon.
Don't be fooled: the skin is a marvelous yet deceptively
difficult and treacherous organ with which to work.
   In my opinion, the irritant reaction is more significant
than the allergic reaction. The obvious, immediate damage
to the skin from chemicals or materials too strong to be
tolerated by anyone requires no elaboration. The subtle,
subclinical irritant reaction which eventually results in
overt gross clinical changes is much more important, elusive,
and common. The oversimplified explanation of chemicals de-
fatting the skin or having toxic effects on proteins and
enzyme systems emphasizes our lack of knowledge in this area.
Fortunately, skin recovers marvelously from numerous minor
insults. Eventually, however, the skin is pushed beyond its
recuperative powers, and symptoms and gross clinical alterations occur. One very common clinical problem is aptly

labeled "detergent burn." Abuse of the skin and its appendages by overcleansing and overexposure to chemicals commonly creates difficulties. Some patch-testing procedures, which are admittedly crude, have been designed to uncover the breakdown of this organ's poorly elucidated protective mechanisms.

An even more difficult but most important area is determination of the frequency of irritation caused by topical agents applied to previously inflamed or diseased skin. Consider the frequency with which cosmetics are used despite the presence of such common problems as seborrheic dermatitis, atopic dermatitis, psoriasis, varicose eczema, sunburn, or miliaria. Just think of using waving solutions and bleaches on skin affected by seborrheic dermatitis or psoriasis. Should a resulting untoward effect be considered solely a reaction to cosmetics? Does the consumer assume the responsibility? What is the responsibility of government and industry? How does one classify such irritations?

Are the stinging and sometimes erythrogenic effects of lotions and creams on xerotic skin and facial seborrheic dermatitis (an oil-rich disorder often interpreted by the layman as dry skin) cosmetic reactions? Aftershave lotion is generally thought ineffective unless some stinging effect follows its use. Is this a reaction? Perception is tempered by custom. Are now a woman's lips dry when she doesn't wear lipstick? Is her face dry when cream is not applied? Why do men not have the same perception when they do not use lubricants on their face? Extend such perception to the consumer who is deciding about reactions to cosmetics.

Allergic reactions may follow a single contact or may occur after many exposures. The whole spectrum of cutaneous changes that reveals the skin's capability to respond is involved in such reactions. Allergic skin reactions to ordinary cosmetics occur only occasionally.

Despite the Westat study of 10,000 families (1), we do not have a good estimate of the frequency of these reactions. The greatest deficiency of that study was its failure to define "reaction." This should have been established much as a judge instructs a jury. And what degree of validation should be required to satisfy the discriminating investigator and those reviewing the figures cited in this study? Would those reported as dermatologist-confirmed reactions stand up in a court of law, especially since the subjects were never seen by a physician? The authority and ability of the reporting person also enter the picture as we evaluate the results of this study. The consumer is the least sophisticated and knowledgeable in interpreting reactions. The physician has more knowledge, but his authority is limited by not having seen the patients and not having better control of the study. The government has the ultimate in influence and power, releasing biased or incomplete information when it wishes. In the eyes of the public, the FDA spokesperson, the President's special assistant for consumer affairs, and more important news releases give stories a label of unchallenged authenticity or credibility. Do the news reporters do their homework or just accept the figures given them? Do we live in a time when the public generally believes and accepts that the government is protecting them? Are there inherent dangers in passively accepting that posture?

THE GOVERNMENT

The governmental agencies have a responsibility in reporting on the cosmetic problem. If they are understaffed, the public should know that. The public also should be informed of exactly what the government does and does not do in trying to police the introduction of products into the market place. How good is the government's continuing surveillance of these products and their advertising claims? How much is being done to disseminate new information about chemicals? What is the interaction between government, industry, consumers, and other interested parties? Governmental agencies should bear some of the responsibility for allowing cosmetics that cause problems to appear on the market and continue to be available. Yet one must realize that those in governmental positions are limited by funds, congressional directives, legal restraints, and scientific information in support of their position.

This creates another type of reaction: the public believes the government has greater capabilities for protection than it really does. Eventually such trust must erode when some unfortunate problem is brought to light, although the government seems to have the unique ability to get itself absolved of responsibility for its mistakes. The great capability of the government to disseminate the news it wants when it wishes to do so is an extraordinary weapon. Whether it is the government's intent or not, its public information frequently is half-truths or unbalanced facts. Ad to this the fact that even the educated public does not read carefully and may be influenced unfairly. But governmental personnel have their own problems in trying to accept their responsibilities and yet handle situations with understanding and temperance. Pressures from consumers, informational services, legislators, and industry, and an innate wish to do a decent job that is entangled in bureaucracy, red tape, and legal constrictions complicate the process tremendously. The difficulty in securing good information from companies, outside scientists, and consumers and in putting all the pieces together with limited facilities and personnel, as well as an explosion in the number of new ingredients, introduces other obstacles. Perhaps the judgment process is under too much stress to allow proper solution and resolution of the difficulties. Guidelines tempered by reasonable judgment have become almost impossible to achieve because of pressure groups and bureaucratic rigidity. For those who seek such direction, preliminary information and general decisions are almost impossible to obtain prior to formulating or marketing a product. Don't these agencies have a conflict of interest when those who vote appropriations inquire about specific situations under agency control? And the agencies must perform and advertise their work to justify continued support.

In the March 1976 issue of *FDA Consumer*, Margaret Morrison wrote about the safety of cosmetics (2). She does acknowledge that some bath soaps and antiperspirants are not technically cosmetics but were included in this study because advertising often emphasizes their cosmetic effects. She further states, "According to the study, a high percentage of the adverse reactions reported by participants was confirmed by dermatologists as being definitely or most probably caused by use of cosmetics." But none of the participants with reactions were seen by dermatologists. In addition she further states, "Since the panel was not randomly selected and the study covered a specific three-month period, the findings cannot be statistically projected to the entire population, or to the annual usage of cosmetics." Nevertheless, "the 35,490 study participants reported 703 adverse reactions that they believed resulted from the use of cosmetics. Of this number, 589 or 84% were confirmed by dermatologists as definitely or most probably caused by cosmetic products." Again, an untrue statement and this one in an official government publication.

THE CONSUMER

The consumer has become sensitized and primed by consumer advocates, action line programs, the government, and similar interested groups. Are we to assume that the public users make the correct diagnosis of cutaneous irritation and allergy from cosmetic items? Obviously, no one knows.

And what about the irritation of skin conditions already present? The frequent occurrence of cutaneous disease, the different physiologic states of the skin, and the changes of temperature and humidity are a few of the more important factors to which the cosmetic-skin interrelationship must

adjust. It is remarkable that the cutaneous envelope copes
so admirably. A high percentage of patients coming to the
dermatologist's office classify seborrheic dermatitis
(dandruff) and eczematous disease as dry skin problems. How
often are these conditions and others irritated by the application of "innocuous cosmetics"? Should such reactions or
untoward effects be charged to the cosmetic companies? In
another sense, cosmetics are basically the vehicles for active therapeutic agents used on the skin, and well-trained
physicians realize that the choice of vehicles is critical
for good treatment. The layman untrained in skin therapeutics may be expected to encounter some problems in selecting
the proper vehicle or cosmetic.

Some reactions are inherent in the use of almost any cosmetic material. What is the allowable percentage of reactions
for any particular formulation? To evaluate this, some
assessment of the importance of cosmetic and toiletry items
to society is needed. However, relatively little hard information exists in this area, which is complicated by misuse
of the product, the refusal or inability of the consumer to
read and understand directions, and the confusion with label
language and technical words. Patients continue to use
preparations to which they are allergic because they feel
they need these items in order to be acceptable in their
society. Should this problem be charged against the companies and physicians or against our social and educational
system? Are our proposed solutions to the problems planned
just for the educated and sophisticated?

Absolute assurance about safety is unreasonable. Without
question, all cosmetics should be made as safe as possible
for those who wish to use them. Society has set certain
standards for social acceptance accruing from the use of
cosmetics. I will not discuss the way in which society
determines these standards. We speak of the benefit-versus-
risk ratio. But maybe this is the wrong approach, since the
word benefit sounds weak in our society. Equals should be
balanced. It should be risk-versus-risk, for is there not a
risk of social unacceptability resulting from not using cosmetics? A step beyond: are we to forbid face lifts, hair
transplants, rhinoplasty, and other similar plastic surgical
procedures? A much more serious risk is present with surgery
than that associated with the use of cosmetics, which I
often think of as a form of bloodless plastic surgery. The
risks, immediate and long-term, should be minimized as much
as possible for all concerned, especially the consumer. Are
not the owners and workers in the cosmetic industry consumers
themselves? The solution should be worked out in a reasonable, cooperative fashion involving all interested parties.
Past mistakes, indiscretions, and outright dishonesty should

not fuel the antagonists.

Finally, the consumer must be fair. Those injured by cosmetics used in a proper way should be compensated adequately, but those deliberately using an item which they know they are allergic to or will cause irritation should assume that responsibility. Labeling will help prevent some of these undesirable effects. The consumer should report significant reactions to the companies and the government. Products causing too many reactions or severe reactions should be removed from the market. Misleading advertising should be stopped and significant penalties should be assessed.

I am assuming the public wants to use cosmetics and toiletry items. If so, they should enter into some reasonable program to ensure that good, safe products are available. Consumer groups may not necessarily represent the vast majority of the public, but they fill a vacuum left by the disinterested and apathetic.

THE PRESS

Freedom of the press is obviously essential in our society. Responsibility for accuracy is essential too. Emphasis on areas that appeal to the reader is acceptable and understandable, but objectivity of reporting still should be the main thrust for all news reporting. Distortion and inaccuracy are all too commonplace.

The publicity on the *FDA Consumer* article (2) on the cosmetic reaction survey discussed above ranged in our area from a prominent story in a Sunday edition of one paper to a small inconspicuous article later in the week in another paper. The information still appears in the press periodically.

Do the reporters understand the question "What is a reaction?" Have they asked for an explanation of the problem which seems so simple but yet is so complex? Even science writers as a group have not asked for clarification or for the divergent views of this situation. Even scientists have much to learn about the intricacies of reactions to materials applied on the skin.

The communications media greatly influence the general public. Each of us at this meeting represents a different spectrum of knowledge and sophistication, but each relies on a clear, honest explanation of our problems, particularly if one is to be an informed consumer. How unfortunate that such a powerful educational force in our society is not used with greater responsibility.

Another type of reaction follows dissemination of news.

Reactive forces are stimulated in all segments of our society. Even some of the scientific news media can be criticized for not asking the spokespersons for elaboration of their views. What does the physician-scientist really mean? Does he have hard evidence to support his statements? What do others think of the material presented? Statements have been made about allergic reactions to parabens, lanolin, perfumes, and other ingredients. How many reactions have occurred? What percentage is represented? How severe are these reactions? Biased or incomplete news statements and advertising copy may lead to the use of unknown and lesser tested materials with greater associated risks.

The inquisitive, fair, and complete mind would result in better media coverage. The dermatologist-scientist, who is supposed to be a more sophisticated cosmetic consumer, frequently falls prey to dissemination of inadequate information. If one hears the half-truths often enough, they become believable. Such a mental reaction may be more damaging than the actual skin reactions to specific products.

No one has a monopoly on truth. Perhaps more questions should be asked than answers given. The authority of the reporter and the spokesperson's stature are most important.

I reported on surveys of dermatologists about cosmetic reactions at this meeting in 1968 and at the American Academy of Dermatology meeting in 1972 (3, 4). It is interesting that the responses reflected the information that was current in the medical press and/or advertising thrusts at the time. If antibacterials in soaps are in the news, they are reported to be the troublemakers. When parabens and preservatives are discussed, they replace antibacterials as the troublemakers. Preconception is obvious in the answers. In addition, bias is present as soon as judgment is involved.

THE COSMETIC INDUSTRY

Tremendous differences exist among the various cosmetic companies with respect to their scientific capabilities, internal structure, and other resources. In contrast to the large company with well-equipped laboratories, the small cosmetic companies may not even know what the government expects of them; they may not receive the *Federal Register* or have anyone in the organization able to read it and give advice. It is difficult also for the small firms to deal with outside testing companies and consultants because of lack of funds and company sophistication. Few, if any, smaller companies are represented at this meeting.

It is necessary that the cosmetic industry scientists not be subservient to sales and promotions campaigns planned by their own firms. Certainly, the promotional material should have scientific validity. The fact that the companies are competitors creates problems in the exchange and handling of information, including reactions to products. In addition, no association exists that can censure those who do not comply within a reasonable framework of acceptable action. Industry efforts reflect our American system of putting out brush fires and patchwork attempts to resolve our problems.

But what is a reaction as seen by industry? We are in need of definitions. Is the stinging of an aftershave lotion a reaction if it is transitory and does not cause a dermatitis? Should we accept overkill and have every conceived deviation reported as a reaction? In addition to definitions, the gradations or importance of reactions should be established as well as the collection of numbers. Should acceptable reactions be only those confirmed clinically or even beyond by a physician? Is an unconfirmed consumer complaint as acceptable as another figure in the total count of reactions? Is this balanced by reactions, confirmed or otherwise, experienced by cosmetic users who merely substitute other products and never report their difficulties? Has the concern about consumer legal action or government intervention resulted in poor handling of the reaction problem? Has the government advertised adequately to get proper registration of companies and reporting of reactions? Regulations are too numerous and complicated and are issued by too many agencies. Many times the requirements are conflicting. Professional legal direction is too costly for many companies. Some companies do not know they are supposed to report reactions to their products. These topics were covered during a conference on cosmetic legislation in Washington several years ago (5).

Control of their own industry and its relationship with the public and government is essential for cosmetic manufacturers and distributors.

STATISTICS AND TEST GROUPS

The numbers game has always been treacherous. The planning and evaluation of studies are most difficult, especially when they involve biological problems. Numbers, tables of numbers, and computer printouts tend to be disarming. Unless these numbers which give the appearance of absolute value are questioned, the information may be misleading.

In the world of biology, a critical look at studies reported 10 to 30 years ago reveals how frequently the numbers do not tell the story accurately. I read little about the frequency of exposure, the relative anticipated risks of

the products, the use on abnormal skin, and the possibilities for misuse. Any why are soap and antiperspirants, which
are not cosmetics, used to produce biased results in a
study (I did it myself in a small survey of dermatologists)
publicized to the entire country? Were all products used as
directed by the instructions on the label?

SUMMARY

   In this report more questions have been raised than
information generated about reactions to cosmetics. Every
way to minimize risks for those who wish to use cosmetics
should be explored. As a start, we need to know "What is a
reaction?"

REFERENCES

1. Westat Study (1975). An investigation of consumers'
    perceptions of adverse reactions to cosmetic products.
    Final report, June, 1975. Commissioned by the U. S.
    Food and Drug Administration.
2. Morrison, M. (1976). Cosmetics: Some statistics on
    safety. *FDA Consumer*, March, p. 14.
3. Lazar, P. (1969). The clinician and reaction to
    cosmetics. *Toxicol. Appl. Pharmacol. Suppl. 3*, p. 1.
4. Lazar, P. (1972). Reactions to cosmetic and toiletry
    items. Presented at Symposium on Cosmetics, 31st
    Annual Meeting Acad. Derm., Bal Harbour, Fla., Dec. 2-7.
5. American Medical Association Conference on Cosmetic
    Legislation (1974). Washington, D.C., March 10-12.

Practical and Theoretical Considerations in Evaluating Dermal Safety

Dorothy B. Hood

Haskell Laboratory for Toxicology and Industrial Medicine
E. I. du Pont de Nemours and Company
Newark, Delaware

Growth in the field of dermal toxicology has been directed largely by the need of various groups to solve their own particular practical safety problems. As a result, some areas of the field have been thoroughly investigated, while others of importance have been touched on lightly or perhaps neglected entirely. Broader knowledge is needed not only to assess dermatitis potential and risk, but often as supporting evidence in resolving a dermatitis complaint in which the problem was not caused by chemical exposure. In addition, if the level of routine testing is to be raised to the more imaginative test design appropriate to the problem at hand, it is essential that the structure and function of the skin as well as the chemical and physical properties of the test material be taken into account.

The purpose of this report is not to give a detailed analysis of test methods, but rather to review relevant biological principles, to focus on some inconsistencies and limitations in the methodology being used, and to make suggestions for improvement.

BIOLOGICAL FACTORS

In extrapolating animal skin test data to likely effects in man, structural differences of the skin should be considered.

Epidermis

The concept of the stratum corneum, a nonviable highly keratinized membrane, as the primary barrier to the passage of foreign chemicals into the vascular system has been established in excised skin and more recently *in vivo*. Although the structure and function of the thicker stratum corneum in man have been well studied, the thinness of the layer in animals and its structural weakness have limited its study in other species. However, it is well to remember in extrapolating data derived from shaved skin of animals to effects in man, that some of the protective capability in animals is normally handled by the hair cover, and the epidermis is correspondingly thinner.

Dermis

Another major difference between animal and human skin lies in the vasculature. It is profuse in man, necessitated by the human skin's thermoregulatory function, and the lymphatic system is also more intricate in man, factors which probably account for the qualitative and quantitative differences in the more highly involved reactions in human skin. Cutaneous reactions to chemicals in man must also be evaluated against the likelihood of lesser penetration.

Transport across the Skin

Although our knowledge of structural differences among species is limited, progress has been made in our understanding of transport of some chemicals across the skin, both excised and *in vivo*. On the basis of these studies, certain species can be ranked in order of skin permeability.

Tregear (1) performed *in vitro* studies with aqueous solutions, organic solvents, solids and highly polar compounds. He then ranked the species in order of decreasing permeability, as follows: rabbit, rat, guinea pig, and man. Bartek *et al.* (2), on the basis of *in vivo* studies with tagged chemicals, ranked them rabbit, rat, pig, monkey, and man, not essentially different.

Franz (3) then tested the Bartek chemicals *in vitro*. Using a single-chamber method he applied the chemicals to the epidermis under ambient conditions. He was able to rank the 12 chemicals in the same order found *in vivo*, although there was considerable variability in the test results. Shaw and co-workers (4) have found good agreement for epinephrine and scopolamine between *in vitro* and *in vivo* tests.

The results of these studies comparing transport across the skin of various species are most encouraging and it is hoped that additional studies will be forthcoming on chemicals of varying structure, until the advantages and limitations of *in vitro* studies are adequately defined and their potential for screening purposes is assessed (5).

Metabolism in the Skin

Perhaps one of the more neglected areas of research pertains to the chemical reactivity or biotransformation of chemicals within the skin. Other than occasional tracer studies, tentative suggestions as to what may occur are usually based on knowledge of the reactivity of the chemical and whether the reactions are less than would be expected from the structure of the chemical. For example, studies of the kinetics of isocyanate reactivity have shown the aromatic isocyanates to be more reactive than the aliphatic. 2,4-toluene diisocyanate reacts quickly with water to form the highly insoluble urea derivative, which could account for the minimal incidence of skin sensitization reported, although it has been shown to be a strong sensitizer when given intradermally to guinea pigs and in the maximization test where barrier function is reduced. Aliphatic isocyanates react much more slowly and tend to produce strong sensitization reactions when applied epicutaneously. Presumably more of the isocyanate is absorbed intact.

Also of current interest is the biotransformation of chemicals by enzymes in the skin. Alvarez *et al.* (6, 7) have shown that skin, like liver, contains an enzyme system that hydroxylates benz(α)pyrene and that the aromatic hydrocarbon hydroxylase activity could be induced by adding benz(α)anthracene to the incubating medium. Human skin showed a lower basal level than rodents, but higher inducibility. Bickers *et al.* (8) have shown the rate to be markedly increased by the presence of DDT and polychlorinated biphenyls. A knowledge of the nature of other metabolizing enzyme systems in the skin would be helpful in designing appropriate toxicological skin tests.

METHODOLOGY

Basic research and new methodology are coming largely from academic institutions with some input from a few industrial organizations. Large-scale screening, however, is being done primarily by industry or by contract laboratories. Potential low-grade irritancy and sensitization are of prime concern to the cosmetic and textile fibers industries, whose products have intimate and prolonged contact with the skin. Insecticides and repellants for personal use are of similar concern. Less extensive tests are usually done where the material is irritating and exposure is more casual, but testing must be sufficient to allow recommending appropriate protective measures.

Examination of our data sources points to several factors affecting methodology. First, extensive, in-depth studies to evaluate marginal irritants and sensitizers generally are confined to a small group of chemicals, namely those used in cosmetics, detergents, and fibers. Second, there is a need of further investigations on human skin, particularly with respect to risk evaluation of products containing known mild to moderate irritants or sensitizers. And third, there is a need for improved communication between those doing research and those who, in the course of safety testing, see many unexplored paths.

DIRECT IRRITATION

Direct irritants are still the major cause of contact dermatitis. It is well to question, therefore, how satisfactorily the established irritancy tests are predicting events. On the basis of the biological data discussed earlier, rabbit skin, generally speaking, would provide the least resistance and human skin the most resistance to entering chemicals. It would seem necessary, therefore, to evaluate animal data critically when extrapolating to effects in man.

The most widely used single-exposure irritancy test is based on the Draize rabbit technique (9, 10), or slight variations of it, as shown in Table 1. It has been used to detect mildly irritating to corrosive materials with varying degrees of success. Criticism of the technique includes (i) inability to retain the dose in a well-defined area of skin, hence dose per given area often varies; (ii) variable results due to the degree of tightness with which the animal is wrapped; (iii) making no exception for the corrosive effect of volatile solvents held under occlusion, resulting in solvents which are only mild irritants when used in normal fashion being classified as corrosive; (iv) frequent inability to determine clinically after 72 hr, whether the injury will be reversible and lack of criteria for irreversible injury based on structural changes; (v) the unusual susceptibility of rabbit skin to certain classes of compounds such as hydrocarbons, solvents, and fatty acid derivatives; (vi) lack of definition for materials which combine with the epidermis, producing reactions which look necrotic, but are

TABLE 1

Direct Irritation—Rabbits

Test	Year	Application Via	Occluded by	Hours exposed	No. days
Draize (9, 10)	1944	Gauze	Impervious wrap	24	1
FHSA (11)	1961	Gauze	Impervious wrap	24	1
FHSA, proposed (12)	1972	Gauze	Impervious wrap	4	1
Weil and Scala (13)	1971	Gauze	Impervious wrap	24	1
Phillips et al. (14)	1972	Gauze	Elastic bandage and cloth sleeve	24	21
Steinberg et al. (15)	1975	Gauze	Elastic bandage and cloth sleeve	24	1
			Elastic bandage and cloth sleeve	24	21
Marzulli and Maibach (16)	1975	Direct	Open	24	14

19

often unaccompanied by inflammation and resolve without scarring.

The Draize technique was examined with respect to reproducibility by Weil and Scala (13). The results from the 22
participating laboratories were highly variable, in some
cases ranging from no effect to corrosive for the same chemical. The high percentage of necrotic reactions for the five
fatty acid derivatives tested showed the undue susceptibility
of the rabbit to this class of compounds, since these materials seldom affect human skin.

Although the rabbit irritancy test results have been misleading for certain kinds of chemicals, they have tended to
err on the side of safety, with criticism being directed
more often toward false positive than toward false negative
reactions, an attribute which should not be underestimated
when safety evaluation is the objective.

Repeated exposure tests to detect low-grade irritants
also show variability. Marzulli and Maibach (16) recommended
the open patch for repeated exposure studies (Table 1) on
the basis that Tregear (1) found uncovered rabbit skin permeability to be roughly comparable to that of occluded human
skin. However, they concluded that the degree of correlation of response between animal and human skin varied considerably and was dependent on the nature of the chemical.
Phillips *et al.* (14) found the rabbit irritancy test satisfactory for materials that were strong irritants or not irritating but less accurate with mild to moderate irritants.
Steinberg *et al.* (15), in repeated exposure rabbit studies
at threshold irritancy levels, found reactions to the chemicals they tested under occlusive conditions to correlate
well with those in man, and they observed fewer differences
in response between open and occluded patches at low irritancy concentrations. The differences in results may relate
to the nature of the chemicals tested, as well as to technique.

Irritation tests performed on other species are summarized in Table 2.

Guinea Pig Tests

Some investigators have found open patches on guinea pig
skin to approximate more closely the response of chemicals
in man. Two industrial laboratories routinely use this procedure and find that the results provide a good basis upon
which to evaluate mild to strong irritation and sufficient
data upon which to safely initiate testing on human skin.

Opdyke and Burnett (20) and Opdyke (21) have used the
guinea pig immersion test for 25 years to evaluate irritancy
of aqueous detergent solutions, and have found a very high

TABLE 2

Direct Irritation Tests—Various Species

Investigator	Species	Exposure Method	Patch
Terhaar[a], Fassett (17)	Guinea pig	Topical	Open
Hood et al. (18)	Guinea pig	Topical	Open
Finklestein et al. (19)	Guinea pig, rabbit, rat	Topical and dye injection	
Opdyke and Burnett (20) Opdyke (21)	Guinea pig	Immersion - aqueous solution	
Justice et al. (22)	Mouse	Topical - back	Open
Uttley and Van Abee (23)	Mouse	Topical - ear	Open

[a]T. J. Terhaar, personal communication.

degree of correlation between the results of this test and reactions in man. It is suitable, however, only for water soluble chemicals of low toxicity.

Mouse Tests

Justice *et al.* (22) and Uttley and Van Abee (23) have reported the mouse to be satisfactory. Follow-up on these tests is needed.

Human Tests

Testing for direct irritancy on man has been primarily concerned with marginal irritants. In order to standardize both procedures and interpretation, Kligman and Wooding (24) suggested calculating an IT_{50}, a figure based on the number of days it takes a very mild irritant to produce overt irritation. Lanman *et al.* (25) have reported it to be useful in formulating new cosmetic products, as have MacMillan *et al.* (26). It is not known whether the test has been used in the development of other types of products.

Additional Species Comparisons

Davies *et al.* (27) have reported that chemicals of varying structure, tested in accordance with the FHSA procedure (Table 1), showed the rabbit to be more susceptible to irritation than man and that the mouse and guinea pig reactions were closer to those in man. MacMillan *et al.* (26), in studies with cosmetic ingredients and formulations, have shown the rabbit, guinea pig, and beagle to respond in that order. Comparative studies of greater scope would be helpful.

HYPERSENSITIVITY

In reviewing the development of skin sensitization testing in guinea pigs, one necessarily starts with the work of Landsteiner and Jacobs (28), who in 1935 showed that intradermal injections of low molecular weight chemicals could be used to induce allergic contact hypersensitivity in the guinea pig. Since that time, variations in technique as listed in Table 3 have been introduced to increase the sensitivity of the test and reduce the induction time. The Draize test method is essentially the Landsteiner-Jacobs method with the introduction of a scoring system to make it suitable for large-scale testing.

Fassett (29) turned to topical applications at low exposure levels, and Buehler (30) and Buehler and Griffith

TABLE 3

Contact Hypersensitivity Predictive Tests--Guinea Pigs[a]

Test	Year	Induction			Challenge	
		Route	Skin	No. of treat.	Patch	Test days (total)
Landsteiner and Jacobs (28)	1935	Intradermal		10	(i.d.)	39
Draize et al.[b] (9)	1944	Intradermal		10	(i.d.)	39
Fassett[b] (29)	1951	Topical	Open	3	Open	28
Buehler, Griffith[b] (30, 31)	1965, 1969	Topical	Occluded	1-9	Closed	16-44
Hood et al.[b] (18)	1965	i.d. or topical	Open	9	Open	40
Magnusson and Kligman (32)	1969	i.d. + topical FCA, SLS	Occluded	1	Closed	24
Maguire (33, 34)	1973, 1975	Topical	Occluded	4	Closed	23

[a] SLS = sodium lauryl sulfate; FCA = Freund's Complete Adjuvant; i.d. = intradermal.

[b] Extensive screening use.

(31) increased the sensitivity of the test by using closed patches for both induction and challenge tests, as does Maguire (33, 34). Hood *et al.* (18) used intradermal injections at higher dose levels for the test for sensitization potential on one-half the group of animals, and open topical applications to abraded skin on the remaining half, to provide some indication of risk.

Magnusson and Kligman (32, 35, 36) used an induction treatment consisting of an intradermal injection plus a closed topical patch applied concurrently, with an injection of Freund's Complete Adjuvant (FCA). They also pretreated the skin with sodium lauryl sulfate (SLS) solution.

The usefulness of the Landsteiner test in detecting low-grade sensitizers has been increased, therefore, by (i) using topical applications under occlusion, (ii) increasing the concentrations of the intradermal injections and using organic solvents for water-insoluble materials, (iii) pretreating the skin with sodium lauryl sulfate to weaken the barrier, and (iv) by injecting Freund's Complete Adjuvant, believed primarily to stimulate the immunological response (32). What has not been done is to run comparisons on the various methods to define their advantages and limitations with respect to various objectives in safety evaluation.

The Draize test has been the most widely used test procedure. However, both Buehler (30) and the present author have found their tests (18) satisfactory for low-grade sensitizers and they have been used extensively for large scale in-house testing, with some use by other laboratories. Efficacy has been judged largely by low incidence of complaints from the field.

There are, of course, many disadvantages in standardizing tests while many determining factors are only partially understood, but it would seem timely to carry out a multiple laboratories study, such as the Weil-Scala study, on the irritant test: several tests using basically different procedures could be checked by a number of laboratories. Test chemicals would be chosen on the basis of widely differing chemical structure and physical properties. Much could be learned from such a study; for example, how the tests compare in sensitivity, whether particular types of chemicals are more likely to produce results by one technique or another, a definition of the factors which are most likely to interfere with interpretation of the data, whether use of Freund's Complete Adjuvant gives misleading results with respect to man, and comparative costs in relation to the amount and quality of data feedback which we can obtain from each type of test.

TESTING PROGRAM IN MAN

The primary purpose of the skin testing program in man is to reduce to a minimum the risk of a new product's causing dermatitis (37). At the same time it is important not to ban a useful product which contains a sensitizer that does not penetrate the barrier in sufficient amounts to cause sensitization. It stands to reason that a problem of this complexity ordinarily cannot be solved by a single test. Studies in man entail a program which starts with a careful evaluation of the chemical and physical properties of the material proposed for use and continues through animal screening and a series of human skin tests until the investigator is satisfied that the risk is minimal. The end use determines what is an acceptable risk. For products like fabrics and cosmetics, where skin contact is extensive, it should be negligible. A somewhat greater leeway may be given to products that are used occasionally and where skin contact is limited. With chemicals used in industry the greater risk is controlled by process design and by protective clothing.

Following the guinea pig test, a decision has to be made as to what additional tests should be carried out on human subjects, keeping this testing to a minimum, but consistent with protecting the public as a whole. The following are the most frequently used tests.

Kligman Maximization Test

If the guinea pig test is negative and a question of species difference arises, the Kligman Maximization Test (38-41) can be used. In this test the barrier action is lowered by pretreating the skin with sodium lauryl sulfate solution, and irritant concentrations of the test materials are employed with tight occlusion of the skin under the patches. The procedure is useful in detecting very low-grade sensitizers, but should be used with caution in predicting the effects of products where effective stratum corneum function is the determining factor in degree of risk.

Schwartz-Peck Test

The Schwartz-Peck Test (42-43), later modified by Fleming (44) to include a 6-day induction period under occlusive conditions, is of particular value in testing polymeric materials which may contain small amounts of low molecular weight sensitizing or irritant chemicals which bleed from the polymer slowly.

Shelanski-Draize Test

Because the original Schwartz-Peck test with one 48-hr
induction exposure did not prove very effective in testing
cosmetics, Shelanski and Shelanski (45) and Draize (8)
recommended multiple insults, namely, 10-15 treatments of
24 hr each. Maibach and Epstein (46) found that the sensitivity of the test could be increased by raising the concentration of the suspect chemical.

Risk Evaluation Test

When a product contains a sensitizer, the risk may be
evaluated by specially designed tests to simulate intensive
use conditions.

Use Test

A limited use test is of value when it is carefully controlled and the subjects are of a type to provide accurate
feedback.

Industrial investigators have found that when strong
sensitizers are screened out of a proposed product by the
guinea pig test, and when low-grade sensitizers are formulated in such a way as to discourage skin penetration, the
program described is satisfactory. Evaluating the extent
of risk when a known sensitizer is involved is a less
exact procedure at the present time.

CURRENT NEEDS

Increasing pressure for data on individual components,
as well as formulations, and the need to prove the negative
are pointing to an acute need for people trained in the
cutaneous aspects of toxicology. It is hoped that it will
not be too long before a Ph.D program is developed in de-
partments of dermatology where candidates could spend part
of their time in industry participating in problem-solving
of the type which confronts investigators daily.

In this branch of toxicology, proper interpretation is
dependent on astute clinical judgment. The usefulness of
the data derived, therefore, is often proportional to the
investigator's understanding of the biological factors involved, the chemical and physical properties of the material
he is testing, and his technical experience. Opportunity
for toxicologists already in the field to take standard
courses in skin biology and allergy and to have an opportunity of seeing positive reactions on human skin would be of

invaluable aid.

In addition to training, closer communication among investigators, such as provided at this joint meeting, and among dermatologists, toxicologists, and those responsible for environmental control is becoming essential.

SUMMARY

The increasing need for in-depth cutaneous toxicity information on biologically active materials in the environment suggested a broad review of current testing programs and an attempt to focus on the problems which tend to dilute the toxicologist's efforts. Suggestions for reducing some of these problems are as follows:

1. Reevaluate the testing program in animals and change procedures which result in too little or misleading feedback.
2. Keep sufficient flexibility in the program to insure growth and improvement.
3. Establish a means of storing and collating animal and verified human data so that they can be used to relate structure and physical properties to the most appropriate testing methods.
4. Establish a means of coordinating and disseminating data derived from experience with new test methods.
5. Increase our training capability.
6. Finally, make a concerted effort to keep up communications among ourselves, even though we must work within limitations presented by proprietary information.

REFERENCES

1. Tregear, T. R. (1966). Physical Functions of Skin. New York, Academic Press.
2. Bartek, M. J., La Budde, J. A., and Maibach, H. I. (1972). Skin permeability in vivo; comparison in rat, rabbit, pig and man. J. Invest. Dermatol. 58:114.
3. Franz, T. J. (1975). Percutaneous absorption. On the relevance of in vitro data. J. Invest. Dermatol. 64: 190.
4. Shaw, J. E., Chandrasekaran, S. K., Michaels, A. S., and Taskovich, L. (1975). Controlled transdermal delivery, in vitro and in vivo. In Animal Models in Dermatology, ed. H. Maibach. New York, Churchill Livingstone.

5. Bartek, M. J., and La Budde, J. A. (1975). Percutaneous absorption, *in vitro*. In *Animal Models in Dermatology*, ed. H. Maibach, New York, Churchill Livingstone.

6. Alvarez, A. P., Kappas, A., Levin, W., and Conney, A. H. (1973). Inducibility of benzo[α]pyrene hydroxylase in human skin by polycyclic hydrocarbons. *Clin. Pharmacol. Ther.* *14*:30.

7. Alvarez, A. P., Leigh, S., Kappas, A., Levin, W., and Conney, A. H. (1973). Induction of aryl hydrocarbon hydroxylase in human skin. *Drug Metab. Dispos.* *1*:386.

8. Bickers, D. K., Kappas, A., and Ahares, A. P. (1974). Differences in inducibility of cutaneous and hepatic drug metabolizing enzymes and cytochrome P-450 by poly-chlorinated biphenyls and DDT. *Pharmacol. Exp. Ther.* *188*:300.

9. Draize, J. H., Woodard, G., and Calvery, H. O. (1944). Methods for the study of irritation and toxicity of substances applied topically to the skin and mucous membranes. *J. Pharmacol. Exp. Ther.* *82*:377.

10. Draize, J. H. (1959). Dermal toxicity. Appraisal of the safety of chemicals in food, drugs, and cosmetics. The Assoc. of Food & Drug Officials of the United States, Texas State Dept. of Health, Austin, Texas, p. 46.

11. Federal Hazardous Substances Act (1961). Title 21, Code of Federal Regulations, Part 191 (from *Fed. Regis.*, Aug. 12, 1961).

12. Federal Hazardous Substances Act (1972). Proposed revision of test for primary skin irritants. *Fed. Regis.*, (244), Dec. 19, pp. 27635-27637.

13. Weil, C. S., and Scala, R. A. (1971). Study of intra- and interlaboratory variability in the results of rabbit eye and skin initiation tests. *Toxicol. Appl. Pharmacol.* *19*:276.

14. Phillips, L., Steinberg, M., Maibach, H. I., and Akers, W. A. (1972). A comparison of rabbit and human skin response to certain irritants. *Toxicol. Appl. Pharmacol.* *21*:369.

15. Steinberg, M., Akers, W. A., Weeks, M., McCreesh, A. H., and Maibach, H. I. (1975). A comparison of test techniques based on rabbit and human skin responses to irritants with recommendations regarding the evaluation of mildly or moderately irritating compounds. In *Animal Models in Dermatology*, ed. H. Maibach. New York, Churchill Livingstone.

16. Marzulli, F. N., and Maibach, H. I. (1975). The rabbit as a model for evaluating skin irritants: A comparison of results obtained on animals and man using repeated dose exposures. *Food Cosmet. Toxicol.* *13*:533.

17. Fassett, D. W. (1951). Chemical constitution, electro-chemical, photographic and allergenic properties of p-amino-N-dialkylanilines. *J. Am. Chem. Soc.* *73*:300.

18. Hood, D. B., Neher, R. J., Reinke, R., and Zapp, J. A. (1965). Experience with the guinea pig in screening primary irritants and sensitizers. *Toxicol. Appl. Pharmacol.* *7*:485.

19. Finklestein, P., Laden, K., and Miechowski, W. (1963). New methods for evaluating cosmetic irritancy. *J. Invest. Dermatol.* *40*:11.

20. Opdyke, D. L., and Burnett, C. M. (1965). Practical problems in the evaluation of the safety of cosmetics. *Proc. Sci. Sect. Toilet Goods Assoc.* *44*:3.

21. Opdyke, D. L. (1971). The guinea pig immersion test--a 20-year appraisal. *CTFA Cosmetic Journal* (Fall issue), p. 46.

22. Justice, J. D., Travers, J. J., and Vinson, G. J. (1961). The correlation between animal tests and human tests in assessing product mildness. *Proc. Sci. Sect. Toilet Goods Assoc.* *35*:12.

23. Uttley, M., and Van Abbe, N.J. (1973). Primary irritation of the skin: Mouse ear test and human patch test procedures. *J. Soc. Cosmet. Chem.* *24*:217.

24. Kligman, A. M., and Wooding, W. M. (1967). A method for the measurement and evaluation of irritants on human skin. *J. Invest. Dermatol.* *49*:78.

25. Lanman, B. M., Elvers, W. B., and Howard, C. S. (1968). The role of human patch testing in a product development program. *Proc. Joint Conf. Cosmet. Sci.*, p. 135.

26. MacMillan, F. S. K., Rafft, R. R., and Elvers, W. B. (1975). A comparison of the skin irritation produced by cosmetic ingredients and formulations in the rabbit, guinea pig, and beagle dogs to that observed in the human. In *Animal Models in Dermatology*, ed. H. Maibach. New York, Churchill Livingstone.

27. Davies, R. E., Harper, K. H., and Kynoch, S. R. (1972). Inter-species variation in dermal reactivity. *J. Soc. Cosmet. Chem.* *23*:371.

28. Landsteiner, K., and Jacobs, J. (1935). Studies on the sensitization of animals with simple chemical compounds. *J. Exp. Med.* *61*:643.

29. Fassett, D. W. (1963). *Am. Dyestuff Report*, August 19.

30. Buehler, E. V. (1965). Delayed contact hypersensitivity in the guinea pig. *Arch. Dermatol.* *91*:171.

31. Buehler, E. V., and Griffith, J. F. (1975). Experimental skin sensitization in the guinea pig and man. In *Animal Models in Dermatology*, ed. H. Maibach. New York, Churchill Livingstone.

32. Magnusson, B., and Kligman, A. M. (1969). The identification of contact allergens by animal assay. The guinea pig maximization test. *J. Invest. Dermatol. 52*: 268.

33. Maguire, H. C. (1973). The bioassay of contact allergens in the guinea pig. *J. Soc. Cosmet. Chem. 24*:151.

34. Maguire, H. C. (1975). Estimation of the allergenicity of prospective human contact sensitizers in the guinea pig. In *Animal Models in Dermatology,* ed. H. Maibach. New York, Churchill Livingstone.

35. Magnusson, B., and Kligman, A. M. (1970). *Allergic Contact Dermatitis in the Guinea Pig - Identification of Contact Allergens.* Springfield, Ill. Charles C. Thomas.

36. Magnusson, B. (1975). The relevance of results obtained with the guinea pig maximization test. In *Animal Models in Dermatology,* ed. H. Maibach. New York, Churchill Livingstone.

37. Maibach, H. (1975)(ed.). *Animal Models in Dermatology.* New York, Churchill Livingstone.

38. Kligman, A. M. (1966). The identification of contact allergens by human assay. I. A critique of standard methods. *J. Invest. Dermatol. 47*:369.

39. Kligman, A. M. (1966). The identification of contact allergens by human assay. II. Factors influencing the induction and measurement of allergic contact dermatitis. *J. Invest. Dermatol. 47*:375.

40. Kligman, A. M. (1966). The identification of contact allergens by human assay. III. The maximization test: A procedure for scoring and rating sensitizers. *J. Invest. Dermatol. 47*:393.

41. Kligman, A. M., and Epstein, W. L. (1975). Updating the maximization test for identifying contact allergens. *Contact Dermatitis 1*:231.

42. Schwartz, L., and Peck, S. M. (1944). The patch test in contact dermatitis. *Public Health Rep. 59*:2.

43. Schwartz, L., and Peck, S. M. (1945). Dermatitis from wearing apparel. *J. Am. Med. Assoc., 128*:1209.

44. Fleming, A. J. (1948). The provocative test for assaying the dermatitis hazards of dyes and finishes on nylon. *J. Invest. Dermatol. 10*:281.

45. Shelanski, H. A., and Shelanski, M. V. (1953). A new technique of human patch tests. *Proc. Sci. Sect. Toilet Goods Assoc. 19*:46.

46. Maibach, H. I., and Epstein, W. L. (1965). Predictive patch testing for allergic sensitization of man. *Toxicol. Appl. Pharmacol. 7*, Suppl. 2, p. 39.

Adequately Substantiating
the Safety of Topical Products

Robert P. Giovacchini

Corporate Product Integrity
The Gillette Company
Boston, Massachusetts

Topical drug, cosmetic, and toiletry products come in contact with the body by being rubbed, poured, sprinkled, or sprayed onto the skin, hair, or mucous membranes. An increasing number of novel products utilizing new ingredients, different mixtures of old ingredients, or in new forms, have reached the marketplace. It is inevitable, and entirely proper, that questions be raised as to whether the safety of these products and their individual ingredients has been adequately substantiated prior to marketing.

This discussion will limit itself to two categories of topically applied products: drugs and cosmetics. These must, in turn, be clearly separated. A cosmetic ingredient is by definition intended only to promote attractiveness; it is not intended to affect any bodily function. A drug, on the other hand, is selectively picked for a specific biological activity and effectiveness against a symptom or disease process. The chemical is used in a form and at a dose level which is intended to have biologically therapeutic effects. Some side effects may be expected and the risk of these may be judged against the effectiveness of the drug, the seriousness of the disease, and other therapy already currently available.

DEFINING SAFETY AND TOXICITY

There appears to be a growing belief that if a chemical, in certain concentrations, is shown to be "nontoxic," then it is safe for addition to a cosmetic formulation. On the other hand, if the material demonstrates toxicity, at whatever concentration, it should not be used in a cosmetic product. Neither position is correct because "safe" ingredients can become toxic in a formulation and "toxic" ingredients can become usable under appropriate conditions. Therefore, before we can proceed we must define what we mean by the terms "safe" and "toxic."

The concept of "safety" exists only with respect to the dose, site of application, and concentration of the chemical or product under conditions of use. Only the uninformed and inexperienced discuss or argue for totally safe, nonhazardous, and biologically inert materials, because no such entities exist. Virtually all substances present a hazard under appropriate conditions and concentrations. Thus, "safety" is freedom from unreasonable risk of significant injury under reasonable foreseeable conditions of use. There are no harmless substances; but there are relatively harmless ways and means of using substances. We have defined safety in terms of the probability that the material will not produce significant damage under certain specified conditions. "Hazard," of course, is the reciprocal of safety. The question is how much of any substance is safe, under specified circumstances.

"Toxicity" is the effect on a biological system or organ that occurs when the agent or its metabolites, under testing conditions, has reached the particular organ or system at the appropriate concentration and for the appropriate time to manifest an adverse change. Changing the dose, route, or duration of exposure can diminish or eliminate the toxic effect on the particular system or organ and thus make the agent "nontoxic" under these particular conditions. To this one must add that any chemical may possess, at certain concentrations and with certain routes of administration, other characteristics such as subject idiosyncrasy, allergy, and tolerances. These must also be considered in evaluating the toxicity of a material (1, 2).

INGREDIENT VERSUS PRODUCT SAFETY

It is extremely important to put into proper perspective the differences between determining the toxic potential of an ingredient or product, evaluating the safety margin of that same ingredient or product, and the relationship of these two types of hazard evaluation to human conditions of use. Safety evaluations deal with developing a margin of nonhazard conditions based on the relationship of concentration, exposure intervals, and mode of application as they pertain to human use of the product. In safety evaluation studies toxicological testing techniques are used, but the objective is one of evaluating the proposed ingredient or product at dose levels that, while they may be exaggerated, do bear a direct relationship to the use of the ingredient or product by the consumer.

Some of the confusion that has arisen on the safety-toxicity of ingredients or products has been due in part to the lack of distinction between the two types of evaluation. The fact that any material can, under certain conditions of testing, produce a toxic effect must be separated from the fact that under other conditions of testing such an effect will not be seen. While the toxicologist will speak of safety factors, margins of safety, and toxic potential, others assume that if any toxic effect is seen under any test conditions, regardless of dose or route of administration, the effect can be assumed to occur under chronic low-level exposure if one looks long and hard enough. Unfortunately, these people are forgetting the controlling factors: the dose, the exposure level, the chemical, the route of administration, and the subject involved.

To date, toxicologists have been unable to devise a set of animal or human toxicological, pharmacological, biochemical, or physiological tests which could demonstrate all the possible effects of a new substance or product in humans. Thus, what may be safe for one individual need not necessarily be safe for another. Irritancy and sensitization are but two notable examples of this variability. Even with the proper use of the ingredient or product, many ingredients may have unavoidable, unexpected side effects. Thus, widespread use of the ingredient or product may well produce unavoidable side effects even if the incidence of such effects is zero or extremely low under controlled laboratory animal or human testing conditions (3).

The twofold concern of the toxicologist should be with the toxicity of the chemical ingredient as such, and with the hazard which may attend its inclusion, in small or large quantities, in a total formulation. These two factors are not the same. The first deals with toxicity per se. The second, while it involves toxicological evaluations and judgments, deals with hazard under certain doses, concentrations, modes of application and use.

The toxicity of an ingredient as such may be investigated by giving animals the chemical by an appropriate route, and observing them for toxic manifestations. To

improve the recognition of such properties the dose is increased, the exposure time lengthened, and target organ-dose
related effects noted in a series of animal studies. From
these studies, preliminary toxicological judgments are made.
Some toxicologists compare therapeutically effective doses
on a body weight basis and toxic dose effects on a surface
area basis. Even here, as for example in oral toxicity testing, one must be careful, because even though a chemical may
be pharmacologically nontoxic, there will be some dose
above which it will affect the laboratory animal simply because of interference with the nutritive intake rather than
because of inherent toxicity (4).

Similarly, materials with low acute toxicity may produce
adverse effects when used repeatedly. Thus, subchronic
evaluation, at appropriate dose levels, is necessary. In
addition, changes occurring in tissues which are not related
to dose level are not necessarily important to the final
toxicological evaluation of the material. While they should
be noted, they should not become a controlling factor.
Lastly, when no toxic effects are seen at responsibly exaggerated doses, additional studies to determine why are not
necessarily required. The fact that a chemical has produced
a toxic effect does not automatically confer extreme hazard
classification to that chemical. While one needs to know
the toxic potential of the individual ingredient, one must
also evaluate the final product at dose levels which bear
some reasonable relationship to the ultimate use of the product. When careful, well-controlled studies demonstrate no
effect, further assumption of hazard should not be considered just because some other study, whose objective was
to prove an effect irrespective of dose, demonstrates a
toxic effect.

There is, therefore, a fundamental but often misunder-
stood difference between these two different aspects of
toxicological testing. The objective of ingredient testing
is to delineate all the toxicological parameters possible
and to demonstrate, irrespective of use, the chemical's
biological activity. The objective of product prognostic
safety testing is to assess hazard under foreseeable conditions of use.

DETERMINATION OF SAFETY

In order to make the determination that a new product
is safe for its intended use, one must review: (i) the
known toxicological information on each specific ingredient,
(ii) interactions between ingredients, (iii) purity and
standardization of ingredients, (iv) the volume and concen-

tration of each ingredient, (v) the method of dispensing, (vi) the directions for use and the dose for use, and (vii) the extent of proposed human exposure. Therefore, one can basically divide the toxicological examination for a topically applied product and its ingredients into: (I) the safety of the specific ingredients and (II) the safety of the proposed new product under (a) toxicological testing conditions and (b) simulated conditions of use.

Since under appropriate laboratory testing conditions all substances can be made to produce toxicological effects, and since we have no set of pharmacological-toxicological tests which will demonstrate all the possible effects of a new substance or product on the human, one cannot follow a "cookbook" set of protocols to evaluate safety, in spite of the attractiveness of this approach. One must instead design a series of studies which best fits the particular product and its particular possible problems.

There is a tendency, undoubtedly for well-intentioned reasons, to assume that substances which are closely related chemically have similar toxicological properties. While this is often true, it is not universally true. Toxicological evaluation by analogy, therefore, can be misleading. Similarly, just because a chemical or product can produce certain effects when orally administered does not mean that the same material will produce the same effect when topically administered. Once any substance or product is inhaled, ingested, or topically applied and absorbed, it will become involved with the intricate chemistry of the body. Some substances will have essentially no effect, and some may produce transient effects based on the body's ability to adapt, while others may produce functional, biochemical, or structural effects which may in turn produce other direct or indirect effects, for example, inhibition of a body defense mechanism.

One cannot look at a list of ingredients and decide if each is or is not acceptable for use in a given product or category without some knowledge of the toxicity of the individual ingredients. In many cases, significant toxicological differences are found that could change the safety of the entire product. Thus, a literature review of the ingredients and a review of the possible chemical interactions between mixtures of ingredients, as well as other considerations and information, are necessary prerequisites to a safety evaluation that is required to ensure the safety of a particular product.

There are many ways in which one may classify potential sources of toxicity. One can list them according to chemical structure, organ or systemic target effect, or characteristics of exposure. In addition, one can subcharacterize

exposure by either acute, subchronic, or chronic use. One
can further break them down into dose and response and,
from this, develop dose-response relationships. One can
break materials down into their chemistry, metabolic and
biological effects, or other factors such as type of vehicle, presence of adjuvants and physical form, as well as
dose, concentration, and route of administration. Finally
there are other factors which relate to the test subjects,
such as species, strain or race, age, sex, nutritional,
genetic, hormonal, immunological status, existence of disease, and environmental factors that include chemical,
physical, and social components.

TESTING FOR SAFETY

There are a large number of measures of toxic effects,
and from them one must develop realistic guidelines to determine the safety of the product in use to avoid injury to
man. In spite of all this, of course, no amount of experimental study can guarantee absolute safety from harm for
any substance. These guidelines are nothing more than
toxicological investigations that provide the data on which
to base a reasonable projection and prediction about conditions under which the product can be safely used. Thus,
the safety projections are never firm, fixed, or unchange-
able. Rather, they represent the best judgment, at any
given time, of the safety of a material based on the sum
total of all the currently available toxicological information (5).

In preparing to substantiate the safety of a proposed
new topical product one must look at the following factors:
1. Chemical composition of the sample to be tested:
    a. active ingredient
    b. vehicle (effect of excipients)
    c. purity of ingredients
    d. stability
    e. physical/chemical characteristics of ingredients
        (particle size, solubility)
2. Exposure conditions and their possible biological
    effects:
    a. dose
    b. volume
    c. concentration
    d. route of exposure
    e. frequency of administration
    f. rate of absorption
    g. duration of exposure
    h. species

     i. number of animals per test group
     j. type of controls
     k. measurements
         i. weight
        ii. appearance
      iii. hemograms
       iv. clinical chemistry
        v. urinalysis
       vi. gross pathology
     vii. histopathology
     l. special studies:
         i. teratology
        ii. mutagenicity
        ii. carcinogenicity

TOPICALLY APPLIED DRUGS

    Earlier, we separated drugs from cosmetics because a drug contains an active ingredient that is intended to be pharmacologically active. Considering the use and activity of the test material, let us look first at the problem of substantiating the safety of topically applied drugs.

    The traditional approach that has evolved for evaluating pharmacologically active materials involves pharmacological studies in animals and then toxicological tests with animals by all possible routes, at exaggerated doses, for both short and long periods of time, in which the animals are subjected to a battery of clinical chemistry and metabolic fate studies. At the conclusion of these tests the animals are sacrificed and all organs are examined for histopathological alterations. Since we are dealing with topically applied products, one must evaluate the potential for local irritation, systemic absorption, and metabolic fate, and the effect of the chemical on inflamed and/or diseased tissue. In addition, if the product is in aerosol form the possible incidental inhalation of the drug when sprayed topically must be considered. Because all possible routes of administration are used in these types of studies, absorption of the material following oral, intravenous, or intraperitoneal application may demonstrate different toxicological potential. One must clearly keep in mind, in reviewing the results of the studies, the proposed final use of the drug. For example, one must distinguish between toxicity by a route of administration not intended for the product and toxicity resulting from the proposed use of the product. Obviously, for topically applied products one must look not only at the potential for skin irritancy, but also at the potential for ophthalmic irritancy, mucous membrane irritancy, and the potential for human irritancy, sensitization, or photoallergic reactions (6, 7).

In summary, when determining the safety of a topically applied drug one must look at the chemical and physical characteristics, the pharmacological activity, the absorption, distribution, metabolism, and excretion of the material, the potential for interactions, and the potential effect on the organ systems. The measures of these potentials are determined through acute, subchronic, and chronic toxicity studies in conjunction with studies to evaluate the potential for skin, ophthalmic, and mucous membrane irritation, sensitization, and photoallergic reactions.

TOPICALLY APPLIED COSMETIC PRODUCTS

In substantiating the safety of a topically applied cosmetic product animal screening studies similar to those described earlier are used. They are: (i) oral toxicity, (ii) ophthalmic irritancy, (iii) percutaneous toxicity, (iv) dermal irritancy, (v) sensitization studies, (vi) photoallergic studies, and (vii) inhalation studies if the product is an aerosol. To substantiate the safety of a proposed new product one should have reviewed the toxicological profile of the various ingredients, the potential for chemical interactions among the various ingredients, the proposed amount and extent of human exposure, and the mode of application. Studies on the proposed new product should be performed on the final formulation for which adequate ingredient and preservative specifications have been established. The final formulation should be reviewed to determine conditions under which foreseeable accidental misuse could result in injury, and whether antidotal measures are required.

In developing the safety substantiation for a particular topical cosmetic the following should be considered. One should determine the potential for skin irritancy, sensitization, photodermatitis, ophthalmic irritancy, and oral and percutaneous toxicity. For products subject to contact with mucous membranes one should also determine the potential for mucous membrane irritancy and absorption. For products in the aerosolized form one should, in addition, consider the potential for toxicity by inhalation. Where the product is used on a repeated basis, the potential for chronic toxicity should also be considered (8, 9).

Are such studies required for every variation of an existing line of cosmetic products? Not necessarily. Where one has already obtained published or unpublished toxicological test data on individual ingredients and on product formulations having similar compositions and use to the product in question, then only those tests, if any, which are appropriate to complete the safety substantiation profile are necessary. In addition, extensive marketing of a product over a long period of time without significant adverse product experience is excellent evidence of safety under conditions of use and, in the absence of other adverse data and information, may be sufficient to show that a product is free from unreasonable risk of significant injury under reasonable foreseeable conditions of use. If additional studies are deemed necessary, then those studies, on animals or humans, that are to be performed must be relevant to the mode and frequency of use of the cosmetic product and to the sites of the body which the cosmetic may reasonably reach.

It would appear that it may always be necessary to examine for evidence of dermal irritation or allergic reactions. It may also be necessary to examine for evidence of systemic toxicity where the product has the potential to be absorbed through the skin or mucous membranes or has the potential for inhalation or ingestion (10, 11).

When should one test for mutagenesis, teratology, or carcinogenesis? All chemicals for which a mutagenic, teratogenic, or carcinogenic hazard cannot be ruled out with reasonable confidence on the basis of expert toxicological judgment should be tested. For example, chemicals whose structure and biological activity resemble those of known carcinogens, or which may form metabolites similar to those formed by known carcinogens, should be tested. Obviously, chemicals that affect rapidly growing tissues and mitosis should be examined. Materials that chemically, biologically, and pharmacologically relate to known or suspected mutagens should be examined, as well as materials that show depression of hematopoiesis, spermatogenesis, and oogenesis, stimulate or inhibit growth of organs, cells or viruses, or inhibit the immune responses. Compounds belonging to a new chemical class for which no apparent information is available, including widespread use, should also be examined by such tests. Unfortunately, in this immensely complex area more knowledge, rather than more advocates, regulation, or politics, is required. Until this knowledge is obtained reasonable questions concerning hazard must be taken seriously, and if they are not resolvable on the basis of existing data a conservative approach must be adopted in order to protect the public. Further, as scientists we must be constantly alert to new techniques which may elucidate and hopefully speed up the time it presently takes to run some of these studies. However, irrespective of speed, cost, or huckstering by particular advocates we must adhere to the postulates of responsible science, originally described by Koch, before we grasp at a new technique or testing protocol (12-16).

SUMMARY

The ultimate goal of substantiating the safety of a topically applied product is to ensure that the product will be safe for the consumer under the recommended and reasonably foreseeable conditions of use. The responsibility for ensuring adequate substantiating of safety rests with the toxicologist. He must be constantly prepared to examine the reasonableness of new safety questions as they arise. He must carefully separate suspicion of toxicity from evidence of toxicity under the conditions of human use. Competent scientific data, documentation, and judgment are the only adequate and technically correct approaches for adequate substantiation of safety. It is the ethical, moral, and business responsibility of each company to ensure, prior to marketing, that it has adequately substantiated the safety of its product.

REFERENCES

1. Hayes, W. I. (1972). *Essays in Toxicology*. New York, Academic Press.
2. Loomis, T. A. (1968). *Essentials of Toxicology*. Philadelphia, Lea & Febiger.
3. Litchfield, J. T. (1965). Predictability of conventional animal toxicity tests. *Ann. N.Y. Acad. Sci. 123*:268.
4. Paget, G. E., and Barnes, J. M. (1964). Toxicity tests. Evaluation of drug activities. In *Pharmacometrics*, eds. D. R. Laurence and A. L. Bacharach. New York, Academic Press.
5. Spinks, A. (1965). Justification of clinical trial of new drugs. In *Evaluation of New Drugs in Man*, ed. E. Zamais, pp. 7-19. New York, Macmillan.
6. Lehman, A. J. (1955). Procedures for the appraisal of the toxicity of chemicals in food, drugs, and cosmetics. *Food, Drug, Cosmet. Law J. 10*:679.
7. Zbinden, G. (1964). The problem of the toxicologic examination of drugs in animals and their safety in man. *Clin. Pharmacol. Ther. 5*:537.
8. Giovacchini, R. P. (1972). Old and new issues in the safety evaluation of cosmetics and toiletries. *CRC Crit. Rev. Toxicol. 1*:361.

9. Giovacchini, R. P. (1969). Premarket testing pro-
    cedures of a cosmetic manufacturer. *Toxicol. Appl.
    Pharmacol. Suppl. 3*, p. 13.
10. Eierman, H. J. (1976). Cosmetic safety substantiation;
    regulatory considerations. *Drug Cosmetic. Ind. 118*:32.
11. Schmidt, A. M. (1975). Food, drug and cosmetic pro
    duct, warning statements. *Fed. Regist. 40*(42),
    8912-8929.
12. World Health Organization (1966). Principles for pre-
    clinical testing of drug safety. W.H.O. Technical
    Report 341.
13. World Health Organization (1967). Principles for the
    testing of drugs for teratogenicity. W.H.O. Technical
    Report 364.
14. World Health Organization (1969). Principles for the
    testing and evaluation of drugs for carcinogenicity.
    W.H.O. Technical Report 426.
15. World Health Organization (1971). Evaluation and test-
    ing of drugs for mutagenicity: Principles and problems.
    W.H.O. Technical Report 428.
16. Paget, G. E. (1962). Toxicity tests: A guide for
    clinicians. *J. New Drugs 2*:76.

The Skin as a Target Organ
for Systemic Agents

Jerome L. Shupack

Department of Dermatology
New York University School of Medicine
New York, New York

When one thinks of organ toxicity, the fundamental considerations include those aspects of anatomy, physiology,
biochemistry, and pharmacology which explain and, on
occasion, predict toxic reactions. For the skin as a target
organ such considerations have lagged somewhat for a number
of practical and some not so practical reasons. It is said
that cutaneous toxicity is rarely life-threatening, nor does
it pose, in most instances, serious long-term morbidity. By
being on the surface, skin is visible, so it doesn't have
the air of mystery of the internal organs such as brain,
kidney, or blood. Most think of the skin as a passive en-
casing membrane, conveniently excluding noxious materials
and preventing the escape of vital body fluids. Such views
continue to pervade the thinking of the faculties of many
medical schools and graduate programs, so that the teaching
of cutaneous biology is relegated to a minor status and many
fertile minds are turned to the more glamorous fields of internal medicine, surgery, and their various subdivisions.

Such views are far from the truth, as I will attempt to
demonstrate. Cutaneous toxicity can be a serious medical
problem. The skin is a fascinating organ with a complex
biology and its accessible location makes it ideal for basic
biologic studies.

GENERAL CONSIDERATIONS

By common consent, the skin includes the tissue that
covers the body, together with certain semimucous and mucous
membranes such as the lips, conjunctivae, nares, external
auditory canals, gingival and buccal mucosa, vulval and anal
canal, as well as the modified cutaneous structures--hair
and nails. Considered as an organ, the skin is impressive
in size and is essential to life. The average surface area
of the skin in an adult male is approximately 20 square feet.
Its weight of 9 or 10 pounds is exceeded only by the muscu-
loskeletal system. The skin of a flayed human adult would
amount to 3.6 liters in volume. Of great importance is the
variation in structural details of skin from site to site in
the body, with corresponding biochemical and functional differences as well as differences of the skin with age, sex
and race.

The skin comprises three major layers: the epidermis,
the dermis, and the subcutaneous fat. The epidermis is
relatively thin, an average figure being 0.1-0.2 mm. The
dermis is approximately 10-20 times thicker, with an average thickness of 2 mm. The upper dermis consists of loose
connective tissue and has projections known as dermal
papillae which interdigitate with the epidermis. There is
a distinct basement membrane separating the epidermis and
dermis. There are superficial arteriolar and venular plexi
as well as neural elements present in the upper dermis and
extending into the papillae. One may also see specific
sensory receptors in the superficial dermis such as the
Meissner corpuscle or the mucocutaneous sensory structure.
The deeper dermis consists of broader bundles of collagen,
running for the most part parallel to the skin surface. In
this area, one may find the eccrine and apocrine sweat glands
with their ducts extending to the surface. In the deep
dermis and sometimes extending into the subcutis one also
finds the hair follicle. Entering the hair follicle approximately two-thirds of the way up is the sebaceous gland.
There is often a smooth arrectores pili muscle that attaches
to the hair below the entrance of the sebaceous gland. Within the dermis are always numerous cells of the lymphocytic,
histiocytic, and fibroblastic types. Separating the dermis
and subcutaneous fat is the deep vascular plexus of the
skin. The subcutaneous fat is of variable thickness and is
composed mainly of fat storage cells and a fine vascular
network. One occasionally sees here the Pacinian corpuscles,
which are end organs mediating sensations of pressure.

The epidermis itself consists of four basic layers:
(i) a basal or germinative cell layer, (ii) the spinous or
prickle cell layer, (iii) the granular cell layer, and

(iv) the keratin layer or stratum corneum. Within the basal layer are interspersed dendritic cells of neural crest origin, the melanocytes which produce pigment that is injected into the basal cells and prickle cells. The amount of pigment produced by these melanocytes gives the skin its characteristic color. Other dendritic cells, the Langerhans cells, appear to act as epidermal macrophages and are involved in the processing of foreign materials passing through the skin which produce an immune response. There is a gradual metamorphosis of the epidermal epithelial cell into the flattened cells filled with kerato-hyaline granules seen in the granular layer. The granular cell then loses its nucleus and becomes fully keratinized, becoming part of the cornified layers from which it is finally shed. This process takes approximately 4 weeks. About 1% of the epidermal cells are lymphocytes and these are probably involved with the immune functions of the skin. The skin is receiving renewed interest as a site for primary immune interaction between external antigenic material and the ever-present population of lymphocytes and histiocytes in the epidermis and dermis. In addition to a neutralizing effect, sensitization and hyposensitization or tolerance phenomenon can occur in the skin, with systemic implications, as we shall subsequently note.

Having thus briefly reviewed the components of skin, it is safe to say that examples are known where practically any and all of these distinct structures may individually be the target for systemic agents. But how specific a target is the skin? When we see a cutaneous reaction, are we seeing a visible manifestation of a systemic response such as a vasculitis, or are we seeing a reaction which can occur only in skin by virtue of some unique anatomic or biochemical feature such as with an allergic contact eczema or certain hyperpigmentation reactions?

When a pharmacologist looks at a systemic agent, there is a fundamental paradigm inherent in all considerations. This relates to the processes of absorption, distribution and protein binding, metabolism and clearance or excretion. These processes are relevant to the organism as a whole or in relation to a specific organ or tissue. Each of these processes is subject to several modulating effects. Individuals of different genetic constitution will react differently to the same systemic agent, so that heredity is sometimes important in understanding a particular effect in a particular individual. The environment, composed of varying combinations of temperature, humidity, irradiation, microorganisms, and chemicals may determine the final effect of a systemic agent in any individual. Lastly, each of us is subject to a number of biologic rhythms, inherent in nature, but probably synchronized by outside factors.

Such rhythmic changes may produce a changing pattern of responsiveness to systemic agents. These theoretical considerations all apply to the skin as an organ. Since my subject involves systemic agents I will not dwell on absorption, which has long been the primary area of concern to cutaneous pharmacologists and toxicologists. I would like to spend some time, however, on the subject of metabolism. Let me separate at once the problem of metabolism by microorganisms on the skin surfaces and crevices. I will refer only to metabolism by skin cells per se. For many years, the metabolic role of the liver has been appreciated. The various biochemical oxidative steps of hepatic detoxification or metabolism of systemic agents seem to be largely mediated by an electron transport system with terminal energy transfer carried out by a unique cytochrome called P450 because of its spectral characteristics (1). In the past few years evidence has been gradually accumulating that the skin is capable of carrying out many of these reactions locally. Although not conclusively demonstrated, there is suggestive evidence that skin may contain cytochrome P450.

The hydroxylation of benzopyrene in the liver is a prototypic example of P450-mediated hepatic metabolism. A simple and sensitive assay using preparations of different tissues incubated with benzopyrene, NADPH, oxygen, and magnesium reveals the presence of P450 activity by the synthesis of 3-hydroxybenzopyrene, easily detected by fluorescence spectroscopy. Conney (2) demonstrated a low level of benzopyrene hydroxylase in the skin of rats. This became more apparent if the skin was first painted with methylcholanthrene, a known inducer of P450 activity. Alvarez (3) duplicated these results using benzanthracene, another P450 inducer, in human foreskins. Bickers (4) using polychlorinated biphenyls, which are also potent P450 inducers, was able to show, after application of these compounds to the skin of rats, a direct increase in liver P450 and a suggestive "blip" appearing in skin at 448 nm. This experiment is of particular significance since it measures P450 directly and does not rely solely on a reaction product.

From this, we can see that skin may play a role in transforming topically applied materials or agents reaching it from within by direct biochemical alteration. If this is so, we can no longer be content with an evaluation of cutaneous toxicity simply in relation to the agent administered, but must now give consideration to the metabolites which may be active, and to rates of inactivation. Also, in relation to cutaneous carcinogenicity, it may be that inactive molecules such as some polycylic hydrocarbons may be converted to active carcinogens by the action of skin metabolism.

I would now like to turn my attention to several examples in which the skin acts as a target organ for systemic
agents. These have been chosen primarily to relate to the
theoretical considerations already discussed.

The classic role of skin as a target organ relates to
allergic reactions produced by systemic agents in individuals
who have previously been sensitized by topical exposure. A
large number of chemicals, when applied to the skin, may
elicit in certain individuals an allergic eczematous contact dermatitis (5). When such an individual is subsequently exposed systemically, either by ingestion or inhalation,
to the same or a related chemical, a skin reaction of an
eczematous type may occur, at first most pronounced in areas
that have previously reacted to the external exposure and
subsequently in a more generalized distribution. The inverse, however, does not seem to be true, in that systemic
administration of a chemical appears to have no influence on
later contact sensitization in man. These facts imply that
the skin has a unique role in "processing" externally applied
chemicals to create a state of hypersensitivity. Many have
assumed that conjugation of simple chemicals or haptens to
skin protein creates a complete antigen which then causes
sensitization. Recent work by Baer and Silberberg (6) suggests that the Langerhans cell may carry the antigen to regional lymph nodes where proliferation of specifically sensitized lymphocytes takes place with recirculation to the
skin to cause the clinically observed delayed hypersensitivity reaction. Such concepts are very much in keeping with
teleological ideas of the skin as the protective external
barrier to a hostile world. Also explained by such a
mechanism is the failure of systemic agents to provoke an
allergic eczematous response unless the individual has previously been sensitized, since appropriate "processing" of
the antigen can only take place following external contact.
Why some individuals become sensitized and others do not,
to the same external exposure, is not well understood.
There is some evidence for genetic predisposition. Also,
the quantity of material applied and the length of exposure
seem important. The major differences, however, are unex-
plained and perhaps exist in the realm of differences in
rates of percutaneous penetration or epidermal metabolism
of the topically applied chemicals.

Numerous examples exist of topical sensitizers and immunochemically related drugs that can cause an eruption
upon systemic administration. For example, sensitization
to hydrazine hydrobromide through industrial exposure may
result in an eczematous reaction upon the administration of
the immunochemically related drugs isoniazid, hydralazine,
or phenelazine. Table 1, taken from Fisher (5), shows other

similar combinations of topical sensitizers and systemic eliciters of eczematous dermatitis, where the skin acts as a specific target organ.

A new addition to this list was recently reported by Christensen and Möller (7) of Sweden. They studied a group of 165 women with nickel contact allergy. Of these, 52% had hand eczema, most with the morphology of "pompholyx," a most difficult clinical problem. The hand eczema showed little correlation with occupational or external contact with nickel; however, 12 of the patients were deliberately provoked by either topical contact with nickel or oral administration. Intense handling of nickel objects caused itching but no eruption in 3 of 12 patients. Oral administration, however, of 25 mg of nickel sulfate containing 5.6 mg of nickel metal resulted in flare of the hand dermatitis with a 3- to 16-fold increase in vesiculation in 9 of 12 patients and eruption at other sites in 7 of 12. The theoretical implications of this study are great. The quantity of nickel administered was somewhat in excess of estimates for the average diet, but when one takes into account metal containers and utensils, it is quite possible that many persons do ingest sufficient nickel to provoke and exacerbate chronic hand eczema. Other contact allergens such as cinnamon may result in aggravation of chronic hand dermatitis. Perhaps this often disabling skin reaction could be avoided in some patients if it could be established that flare-ups result from the systemic ingestion of chemicals to which the individual has developed contact sensitivity.

Vitiligo is a condition in which areas of skin become white or pale but otherwise are normal. Extension may be rapid or may proceed slowly and intermittently over many years. The cause is considered unknown. Depigmentation with similar clinical appearance can be caused by certain phenolic detergent germicides, as reported by Kahn (8). The exact mechanism for the effectiveness of these agents in producing pigment loss is not clear, but is probably related to their interference with the biochemical pathway for melanin synthesis by acting as tyrosine analogs leading to the synthesis of abnormal DOPA-like intermediates. Various chemicals of related structure may produce a similar effect. Why certain individuals are affected preferentially is not clear. By analogous reasoning with the example of nickel ingestion exacerbating hand dermatitis in nickel-sensitive patients, could vitiligo be a cutaneous reaction pattern to systemically ingested phenolic compounds or to endogenously formed abnormal catechols? This would seem a fruitful area for research in vitiligo, a disease of unknown etiology.

Heavy metals may produce hyperpigmentation of the skin, presumably by direct deposition in the cutis such as in the

TABLE 1

Topical Sensitizers and Immunochemically Related Drugs that Can Cause an Eruption upon Systemic Administration[a]

Topical sensitizers	Immunochemically related drugs
Hydrazine hydrobromide	Isoniazid, Apresoline, Nardil
Para-amino compounds	Para-aminobenzoic acid (PABA) and related local anesthetics (benzocaine, procaine) Azo dyes in foods and drugs Dymelor, Orinase, Diabinese, sulfonamides Diuril, Hydrodiuril, Saluron, Renese Para-aminosalicylic acid (PAS)
Balsam of Peru	Cinnamon
Neomycin sulfate	Streptomycin, kanamycin
Resorcin	Hexylresorcinal (Crystoids, Caprokol)
Organic and inorganic mercurials	Mercurial diuretics
Metallic mercury	Calomel
Cobalt	Vitamin B_{12}
Thiamine	Coenzyme B (cocarboxylase)
Ethylenediamine hydrochloride	Aminophylline, Antistine, Phenergan, Pyribenzamine, Synopen, Neohetramine
Formaldehyde	Urotropin, Mandelamine, Urised
Thiram and disulfiram	Antabuse
Halogenated hydroxyquinolines	Vioform, Diodoquin

TABLE 1 - Cont'd.

Topical Sensitizers and Immunochemically Related Drugs that Can Cause an Eruption upon Systemic Administration[a]

Topical sensitizers	Immunochemically related drugs
Chlorobutanol	Chloral hydrate
Iodine	Iodides, iodinated organic compounds
Benadryl	Dramamine

[a]Data from A. A. Fisher (5). We thank the author and publisher for permission to use the table.

case with silver and the condition known as argyria. Some, such as arsenic, may favor the synthesis of melanin by sulfhydryl binding. The precise mechanisms, however, for the localization or distribution of metals to the skin are not known in a pharmacologic sense.

Lupus erythematosus is another disease of unknown etiology. Certain drugs, especially those with free amino or hydrazine groups, may produce an iatrogenic form of the disease even with cutaneous manifestations. The metabolism of free amino groups takes place in the liver and blood by an acetylating enzyme, N-acetyl transferase. The activity of this enzyme is genetically controlled so that some individuals rapidly inactivate these drugs and others do so less rapidly (9). For example, if one measures the plasma concentration of free isoniazid remaining after 6 hr of acetylation in a normal American population, two groups are noted: the rapid acetylators, who quickly metabolize the drug resulting at a fixed 6-hr interval in a low plasma level, and the slow acetylators with a residual higher concentration. The proportionate numbers are roughly 50:50. Perry (10) reported that all of his patients who developed lupus-like symptoms following administration of hydralazine were slow acetylators. Reidenberg (11) examined 14 patients with spontaneous systemic lupus erythematosus and found a predominance of slow acetylators different from the expected 50:50 distribution in the population at large.

SUMMARY

The point to be made from this brief discussion of apparently disparate examples in which the skin behaves as a target for systemic drugs is this: to fully appreciate a cutaneous reaction to a systemic drug, one must have an understanding of more than immunology. One must know all aspects of the pharmacology of that drug. In the past, too much was made of morphologic reaction patterns and agents producing similar morphologic responses were thought to act by similar mechanisms. However, not all urticarias are allergic. Not all hyperpigmentation or hypopigmentation reactions occur by the same biochemical mechanism.

Each cutaneous response to a systemic agent must be understood in relation to the pharmacology of that agent, its absorption, distribution, metabolism, and clearance, and in relation to other modifying considerations such as the individual's specific genetic constitution and environment at the time of the skin reaction.

It is only by achieving such comprehension that one can gain a solid structure of understanding of the vast panorama of cutaneous reactions elicited by systemic agents.

REFERENCES

1. La Du, B. N., Mandel, H. G., and Way, E. L. (1971). Microsomal enzyme systems which catalyse drug metabolism. In *Fundamentals of Drug Metabolism and Drug Disposition*, ed. G. J. Mannering, Chapter 12, pp. 206-252. Baltimore, Williams & Wilkins.
2. Schlede, E., and Conney, A. H. (1970). Induction of benzo(α)pyrene hydroxylase activity in rat skin. *Life Sci. (Part II)* 9:1295.
3. Alvarez, A. P., Conney. A. H., Levin, W., Merkatz, I., and Kappas, A. (1972). Induction of benzopyrene hydroxylase in human skin. *Science* 176:419.
4. Bickers, D. R., Kappas, A., and Alvarez, A. P. (1974). Differences in inducibility of cutaneous and hepatic drug metabolizing enzymes and cytochrome P450 by polychlorinated biphenyls and 1,1,1-trichloro-2,2-bis (p-chlorophenyl) ethane (DDT). *J. Pharmacol. Exp. Ther.* 188:300.
5. Fisher, A. A. (1973). Systemic eczematous contact-type dermatitis. In *Contact Dermatitis*, Chapter 17, pp. 293-305. Philadelphia, Lea & Febiger.
6. Silberberg-Sinakin, I., Thorbecke, G. J., Baer, R. L., Rosenthal, S. A., and Berezowsky, B. (1976). Antigen-bearing Langerhans cells in skin, dermal lymphatics and

in lymph nodes. *J. Cell. Immunol. 25:*137.

7. Christensen, O. B., and Möller, H. (1975). Nickel allergy and hand eczema. *Contact Dermatitis 1:*129.

8. Kahn, G. (1970). Depigmentation caused by phenolic detergent germicides. *Arch. Dermatol. 102:*177

9. La Du, B. N. (1965). Pharmacogenetics. *Toxicol. Appl. Pharmacol. 7,* Suppl. 2, p. 27.

10. Perry, H. M., Jr., Tan, E. M., Carmody, S., and Sakamoto, A. (1970). Relationship of acetyl transferase activity to antinuclear antibodies and toxic symptoms in hypertensive patients treated with hydralazine. *J. Lab. Clin. Med. 76:*114.

11. Reidenberg, M. M., and Martin, J. H. (1974). The acetylator phenotype of patients with systemic lupus erythematosus. *Drug Metab. Dispos. 2:*71.

Cutaneous Absorption and Systemic Toxicity

Donald J. Birmingham

Department of Dermatology and Syphilology
Wayne State University School of Medicine
Detroit, Michigan

Substances which cause fatal or at least serious toxic
reactions in man and animals continue to surface from
hundreds of organic and inorganic chemicals such as gases,
metallics, biologic materials, economic poisons, plant toxins,
radioactive substances, and modern medicaments. Most often,
fatal or near-fatal effects have resulted from accidental or
intentional ingestion, inhalation, or injection of the toxicant. Systemic poisoning or intoxication by percutaneous
absorption is conspicuously less frequent; but when it
happens, fatal or near-fatal effects can follow (1).

Anatomically, the skin is a readily accessible exposure
site for foreign substances of all sorts. However, skin
does not generally behave like the lungs or the gastrointestinal tract with respect to the entry of harmful agents.
This apparent difference was recognized many years ago to
the point that Fleisher believed the skin impermeable to all
substances, including gases. Early in this century, his
hypothesis was discarded in favor of evidence showing cutaneous permeability to lipids and gases and impermeability to
water and electrolytes (2). Since then, much has been
learned about penetration routes, identification and measurement following penetration, factors influencing penetration,
and the role of the stratum corneum in cutaneous defense
through work by Rothman, Blank, Scheuplein, Malkinson,
Stoughton, Kligman, and Vickers, among others (3-7).

The effectiveness of any substance in causing systemic toxicity by percutaneous absorption depends upon two unrelated properties: first, the ability to penetrate transepidermally via the stratum corneum epidermal cell layers, epidermal-dermal membrane, with possibly some initial entry by way of the follicular and sweat duct routes and then enter into the circulation; second, the ability to injure a particular target site or other organs after being transported there in the same or in a biotransformed state (1-4).

Cutaneous penetration depends largely upon the clinical nature of the penetrant and is mainly a function of solubility and diffusion. Lipid-soluble compounds as a group are better absorbed than water-soluble compounds. However, if a compound is both lipid- and water-soluble, it will have greater absorbability. Even then, solubility is not the sole determinant because pH, extent of ionization, molecular size, temperature, and humidity also influence the absorption of materials through the skin (2-4).

Skin has the capacity of responding in several different ways, depending upon the nature and dose of the material making contact: (i) it may act as a relatively complete barrier against penetration; (ii) it can react in the form of mild or severe irritation confined to the skin; (iii) it can be severely injured by corrosive chemicals with resultant systemic toxic effects; (iv) it can respond by developing an allergic eczematous contact dermatitis following penetration of the antigenic agent and subsequent development of delayed hypersensitivity; (v) it can serve as a reservoir for delayed release of the contactant (7); (vi) it can fail to barricade the foreign agent which then traverses the skin layers to enter the circulation and cause a systemic reaction. In this latter category reside a number of materials encountered in agriculture, industry, and in therapeutic medicine.

AGRICULTURE

Most agricultural workers are exposed to pesticides of one kind or another. The number who have experienced toxic effects from these substances is not well defined, but during the period 1960-1971 the number of occupational illnesses among farm workers attributed to pesticides in California amounted to 5,500 cases exclusive of eye and skin afflictions (8). Hayes' recent text on the *Toxicology of Pesticides* cites the mortality level from these agents in 1968 as 72 deaths and a morbidity ratio of 100:1 (9).

Pesticides are generally grouped into their intended uses, namely, insecticides, rodenticides, fungicides, and fumigants. They can be further classified into phosphate esters, chlorinated hydrocarbons of various types, and miscellaneous materials of botanical origin or other mixtures composed of organic or inorganic chemicals (9, 10).

Organo Phosphates

Hundreds of compounds reside within this class of pesticidal agents, some of the better known ones being chlorothion, Diazinon, EPN (ethyl-*p*-nitrophenyl-thionobenzenephosphonate), Guthion, malathion, parathion, and TEPP (tetraethylpyrophosphate). Most of the organic phosphates are absorbed through the skin, but vary in penetrability and in toxicity. Their harmfulness rests in their capacity to inhibit cholinesterase, thereby permitting acetylcholine to function in an uncontrolled system. As a result, they overstimulate the central nervous system and all structures innervated by the parasympathetics. For example, the gastrointestinal and respiratory tracts, sweat and salivary glands, urinary bladder, heart, and pupil. Without prompt and adequate treatment, respiratory failure results from central depression and direct pulmonary obstructive phenomena (9, 10).

Chlorinated Hydrocarbons

Chlorinated hydrocarbon insecticides are neurotoxins and include such products as aldrin, chlordane, dieldrin, endrin, heptachlor, lindane, toxaphene, and Kepone. Most of these compounds are fat soluble and frequently are used in solvent vehicles which facilitate entry through skin. Excessive exposure produces central nervous system effects, e.g., anxiety, tremors, ataxia, convulsions, etc. Some of these have been banned as insecticides because of their persistence in the environment (8-10).

Inorganic Chemical Pesticides

Inorganic chemical pesticides include antimony, arsenic, fluoride, thallium, selenium, mercury, and phosphates. All can injure the skin directly, but systemic toxicity by way of skin absorption is less likely than by exposure through inhalation. Other well known chemical pesticides capable of penetrating skin are the cyanides, dinitrophenol, carbon disulfide, and chlorphenols, among others. All have been incriminated in toxic reactions, but it is difficult to state with certainty the major entry site (8-10).

Botanical Pesticides

Botanical pesticides that contain nicotine or pyrethrin or rotenone-nicotine are the most toxic. Tobacco leaves applied to skin have caused poisoning, and nicotine infusions used as enemas to kill parasites have caused fatalities in youngsters (11). Green tobacco sickness, which regularly occurs in North Carolina, is believed caused by absorption of nicotine, but the symptoms can mimic those of organo phosphate toxicity (12). Nicotine stimulates and then depresses all sympathetic and parasympathetic ganglion cells to produce a paralysis of respiratory musculature (1).

Skin exposure during spraying of pesticides varies widely depending upon equipment being used for spraying, protective clothing, and exposure time involved. Measured evidence of skin absorption has been ascertained experimentally by Blank (13), Greisemer (14), Fredriksson (15), and others. More recently, Maibach and Feldman (16) used selected organo phosphate and chlorinated hydrocarbon pesticides labeled with 14C and measured the 5-day excretion following application of specific amounts of the pesticides to the forearms of six adult subjects. All of the test substances penetrated—some in greater amounts than others. Also demonstrated were absorption differences of body sites; for example, absorption capacity was highest for the scrotum, followed by axilla, forehead, palms, and, finally, forearm.

INDUSTRIAL TOXICANTS

Systemic effects from the inhalation of certain industrial chemicals are occurring all the time, though less frequently than in the past. Chemicals known to cause systemic reactions, including fatalities, by way of cutaneous penetration can be divided into four major groups.

Alcohols and Glycols

Among these compounds, ethylene chlorhydrin is a central nervous system toxicant said to be as potent through the skin as when inhaled. It is encountered in organic chemical synthesis, in the dyeing of textiles, varnish and lacquer manufacture, in potato growing, and in some resin compounding.

Aromatic Nitro and Amino Compounds

This grouping includes aniline, nitrobenzene, dinitrotoluene (DNT), and trinitrotoluene (TNT), among others.

Most of these aromatics go through the skin and induce methemoglobinemia. Aniline poisoning is rare, except in industry, where it is considered an essentially reversible process. It has been associated with infant deaths following skin absorption from ink-marked diapers (18, 19). Other information reveals that methemoglobinemia resulted when 3,4,4 trichlorocarbanilide (TCC), used as a diaper rinse, released aniline during sterilization of the diapers being used in hospital nurseries (20).

During World Wars I and II, trinitrotoluene caused deaths and high morbidity among people employed in bomb- and shell-loading plants. Both TNT and DNT are absorbed through skin, but it is most likely that hepatic and hematopoetic toxicity arises more from dust and vapor inhalation as well as accidental ingestion of particulate TNT (19).

Chlorinated Hydrocarbons

Substances such as methyl chloride, methylene chloride, vinyl chloride, ethyl chloride, chloroform, trichloroethylene, and perchlorethylene probably do not penetrate skin in sufficient amounts to induce systemic effects. Similarly, carbon tetrachloride can penetrate skin, but it is less of a toxicant than when inhaled (21).

Chlorinated biphenyls and naphthalenes have produced serious cutaneous and systemic toxic effects. Chloracne and hyperpigmentation are prominent and often persistent cutaneous changes. Hepatotoxicity, sometimes porphyria, and neuropathy reflect serious systemic changes. Several outbreaks of chloracne and liver dysfunction caused by the arachlors, synthetic waxes containing diphenyls, Halowax containing chlorinated naphthalene, and intermediates encountered in the manufacture of 2,4,5T herbicide have been reported (22-24). It is not known how much of the systemic effects are caused by percutaneous absorption as compared to the inhalation route.

Metals

Few of the metal compounds penetrate skin to produce systemic reactions. Boranes are highly toxic substances employed as high energy fuels, in nuclear reactors, in case hardening of steel, and as fire retardants. Both diborane and pentaborane penetrate skin readily; the major action of these compounds is to produce central nervous system toxicity (25).

Mercury is used in great amounts in the electrical, pharmaceutical, and chemical industries because of its versatility. Inorganic and organic vapors and dusts are

readily inhaled, and certain mercurials can penetrate skin
and accumulate to toxic levels. This metal percipitates
protein, has an affinity for sulfhydryl groups, and causes
tubular necrosis of the kidney. Chronic mercurialism reveals itself by the presence of gingivitis, gingival mercury
line, loose teeth, metallic taste, tremors, ataxia, and
mental confusion (26).

Tetraethyl lead is highly toxic and penetrates skin
rapidly to cause encephalopathy. Toxic exposures from inhalation and skin absorption have occurred during preparation
and blending. Systemic intoxication from dispensing gaso-
line containing tetraethyl lead is unlikely (1, 17).

MEDICATIONS

Any number of drugs have caused various degrees of serious reactions following ingestion or injection. The opposite
is generally the rule for topical medicaments. Of course, if
allergic contact eczematous dermatitis is considered an ex-
pression of systemic intoxication, then the number of contact agents capable of inducing this effect is greatly increased. Allergic contact cutaneous sensitization usually
does not constitute a serious or life-threatening situation.
However, such instances have occurred in systemic eczematous
contact-type dermatitis. Considering the number and types
of medications used on the skin, it is evident that the skin
provides a fairly staunch defense against injury by medicaments. None the less, certain topicals have been identified
as causing fatal or at least serious systemic reactions.

Boric Acid

This material was used in irrigant, powder, and ointment
preparations for years and was a common household antiseptic.
It was first noted as toxic following use in peritoneal ir-
rigation. By 1962 there had accumulated some 175 cases of
toxicity, about one-half of which were fatalities in children. Thirty of the deaths occurred from the application of
pure boric acid powder to diaper dermatitis areas. The resultant toxicity appears as a generalized erythema and
desquamation, accompanied by signs of central nervous system
irritation and renal injury including anuria. The desquamation accompanying the toxicity has been described as re-
sembling toxic epidermal necrolysis. Boric acid does not
penetrate undamaged skin, but readily enters open wounds,
burned skin, or active areas of dermatitis (27-29).

Salicylic Acid

Varying concentrations of this substance are used for keratolytic therapy on many dermatoses and for chemical destruction of warts, calluses, and corns. Prior to the advent of most of the presently used topical agents, salicylic acid was employed extensively in the treatment of psoriasis, seborrheic dermatitis, and superficial mycoses, among other dermatologic disorders. A report in 1964 described the toxic action of a topical ointment containing salicylic acid which was used in the treatment of three cases of widespread psoriasis (30). Two of the patients had been treated with 6% sulfur and 6% salicylic acid in Eucerin cream, the other with 3% sulfur and 3% salicylic acid in Eucerin cream. The patients had six ointment applications, two soap and water baths, and ultraviolet light therapy daily. All three developed varying signs of salicylism such as nausea, vomiting, headache, decreased ability to hear, tinnitus, and central nervous system effects by the 4th day of therapy. All showed significant salicylic acid levels in the serum, thus adequately documenting the absorption which can occur through psoriatic skin. Symptoms abated within a day after discontinuance of treatment. The authors briefly reviewed previously published reports in which salicylic acid had caused 13 deaths. Several additional cases of nonfatal salicylism from topical applications have been reported. Certain factors which influence percutaneous absorption, for example, frequency of application, concentration, area of application, degree of hydration of keratin, and the vehicle, were emphasized (30).

Hexachlorophene

This chlorinated derivative of phenol has been in widespread use for several years in hospitals, medical and dental offices, restaurants, industrial plants, and in many conventional deodorant soaps. A few years ago it was found that the chemical caused toxic neurologic changes in rats. Similarly, investigations in a neuropathology laboratory conducted between 1966 and 1972 revealed several cases of encephalopathy in premature and young infants who had been bathed daily with undiluted hexachlorophene (31). Older infants included in the postmortem study did not reveal such changes. The chemical has been adjudged as causal in the deaths of two children with wide-spread ichthyosis and two children with burns. Other instances of systemic toxicity following percutaneous absorption have been reported. Presently it is advisable to refrain from using the material on widespread areas of injured skin or on premature or small infants (32).

SUMMARY

Several chemicals and medications known to have caused systemic intoxication following percutaneous absorption have been reviewed. Additional toxic materials exist in each respective category; however, experimental and clinical documentation of toxicity in humans is meager. None the less, considering the breadth of the spectrum of contactants to which skin is exposed and its response to these materials, it is wholly appropriate to paraphrase a statement by Irvin Blank: normal skin is a good barrier against transport of almost all substances, but a perfect barrier to few.

REFERENCES

1. Arena, J. M. (1974). *Poisoning - Toxicology - Symptoms - Treatment*. Springfield, Ill., Charles C. Thomas.
2. Rothman, S. (1954). *Physiology and Biochemistry of the Skin*. Chicago, University of Chicago Press.
3. Blank, I. H., and Scheuplein, R. J. (1964). The epidermal barrier. In *Progress in the Biological Sciences in Relation to Dermatology 2*, eds. A. Rook and R. A. Champion. Cambridge University Press, Cambridge.
4. Malkinson, F. (1964). Permeability of the stratum corneum. In *The Epidermis*, eds. W. Montagna and W. C. Lobitz. New York, Academic Press.
5. Stoughton, R. B. (1964). Some *in vivo* and *in vitro* methods for measuring percutaneous absorption. In *Progress in the Biological Sciences in Relation to Dermatology 2*, eds. A. Rook and R. A. Champion. Cambridge University Press, Cambridge.
6. Kligman, A. M. (1964). The biology of the stratum corneum. In *The Epidermis*, eds. W. Montagna and W. C. Lobitz. New York, Academic Press.
7. Vickers, C. F. H. (1972). Stratum corneum reservoir for drugs. In *Advances in Biology of the Skin*, eds. W. Montagna, E. J. Van Scott, and R. B. Stoughton, Vol. XII. New York, Appleton-Century-Crofts.
8. *Occupational Exposure to Pesticides*. Report to the Federal Working Group on Pest Management from the Task Group on Occupational Exposure to Pesticides, 1974. Federal Working Group on Pesticide Management, Washington, D. C., U.S. Government Printing Office.

9. Hayes, W. J., Jr. (1975). *Toxicology of Pesticides.*
    Baltimore, Williams & Wilkins.
10. Gibson, R. L., and Milby, T. H. (1964). Pesticides. In
    Occupational Diseases -- A Guide to Their Recognition,
    ed. W. M. Gafafer. U.S. Dept. of HEW. Public Health
    Service Publication 1097, Washington, D.C., U.S.
    Government Printing Office.
11. Polson, C. J., and Tattersall, R. N. (1969). *Clinical
    Toxicology.* Philadelphia, J. B. Lippincott.
12. Gehlbach, S. J., Williams, W. A., Perry, L. D., and
    Woodall, J. (1974). Green tobacco sickness: Illness
    of tobacco harvesters. *J. Am. Med. Assoc. 229*:1880.
13. Blank, I. H., Griesemer, R. D., and Gould, E. (1957).
    The penetration of an anti-cholinesterase agent (SARIN)
    into skin. Rate of penetration into excised human skin.
    J. Invest. Dermatol. 29:299.
14. Griesemer, R. D., Blank, I. H., and Gould, E. The pene-
    tration of an anticholinesterase agent (SARIN) into
    skin. (III. Method for studying the rate of penetra-
    tion into living rabbit skin. *J. Invest. Dermatol. 31*:
    255.
15. Fredriksson, T. (1958). Studies on the percutaneous
    absorption of SARIN and two allied organo-phosphorous
    cholinesterase inhibitors. *Acta Derm.-Venereol. 38,*
    Suppl. 41.
16. Maibach, H. I., and Feldman, R. (1974). Systemic ab-
    sorption of pesticides through the skin of man,
    Appendix B. *Occupational Exposure to Pesticides.*
    Federal Working Group on Pest Management, Washington,
    D.C., U.S. Government Printing Office.
17. Deichman, W. B., and Gerarde, H. W. (1969). *Toxicology
    of Drugs and Chemicals.* New York, Academic Press.
18. Von Oettingen, W. F. (1941). The aromatic amino and
    nitro compounds; their toxicity and potential dangers--
    A review of the literature, P.H.S. Bulletin No. 271.
    Washington, D.C., U.S.P.H.S.
19. Hamblin, D. O. (1963). Aromatic nitro and amino com-
    pounds. In *Industrial Hygiene and Toxicology, II.
    Toxicology,* ed. F. A. Patty, 2nd edition. New York,
    Wiley-Interscience.
20. Cooper, P. (1974). *Poisoning by Drugs and Chemicals,*
    3rd edition. Chicago, Yearbook Publishers, Inc.
21. Irish, D. D. (1963). Halogenated hydrocarbons. In
    Industrial Hygiene and Toxicology, II. Toxicology,
    ed. F. A. Patty, 2nd edition. New York, Wiley-
    Interscience.
22. Kimmig, J., and Schulz, K. H. (1957). Occupational
    chloracne caused by aromatic cyclic ethers.
    Dermatologica 115:540.

23. Jensen, N. E., Sneeden, I. B., and Walker, A. E. (1972). Tetrachlorobenzodioxin and chloracne. *Trans. St. Johns Hosp. Germatol. Soc.* *58*:172.

24. Taylor, J. S. (1974). Chloracne--a continuing problem. *Cutis* *13*:585.

25. Roush, G., Jr. (1959). The toxicology of the boranes. *J. Occup. Med.* *1*:46.

26. Stokinger, H. A. (1963). The metals. In *Industrial Hygiene and Toxicology, II. Toxicology,* ed. F. A. Patty, 2nd edition. New York, Wiley-Interscience.

27. Goodman, L. S., and Gilman, A. (1975). *The Pharmacological Basis of Therapeutics,* 5th edition. New York, Macmillan.

28. Valdes-Dapena, M. A., and Arey, J. B. (1962). Boric acid poisoning. *J. Pediatr.* *61*:531.

29. Skipworth, G. B., Goldstein, N., and McBirde, W. P. (1967). Boric acid intoxication from medicated talcum powder. *Arch. Dermatol.* *95*:83.

30. Von Weiss, J. F., and Lever, W. F. (1964). Percutaneous salicylic acid intoxication in psoriasis. *Arch. Dermatol.* *90*:614.

31. Shuman, R. M., Leech, R. W., and Alvord, E. C., Jr. (1973). Neuropathology in newborn infants bathed in hexachlorophene. *Morbidity and Mortality* *22*:93.

32. Kimbrough, R. D. (1973). Review of the toxicity of hexachlorophene including its neurotoxicity. *J. J. Clin. Pharmacol.* *13*:439.

Factors Affecting Percutaneous Absorption

Frederick D. Malkinson and Louisa Gehlmann

Department of Dermatology
Rush-Presbyterian-St. Luke's Medical Center
Chicago, Illinois

In the human, the skin's physiological function as a protective organ is served by its profoundly effective barrier properties against the penetration of a wide variety of substances. Compared to most other tissues, the surface of the skin is only slightly permeable. Nevertheless, many substances do penetrate intact skin to some degree, and these are absorbed very much more rapidly if the epidermis is diseased or damaged. Environmental and industrial hazards--liquids, gases, and other chemicals--and certain medications may penetrate normal skin and produce local or systemic toxic effects. Consequently, a knowledge of the general principles governing percutaneous absorption, the factors affecting them, and the significance of the transcutaneous route of absorption are all of importance to the toxicologist.

The term percutaneous absorption will be used in this paper to denote passage of substances from the outside through the entire epidermis with subsequent diffusion into the dermis and entry into blood and lymphatic vessels. The factors affecting percutaneous absorption can be best appreciated following a very brief description of the overall principles governing cutaneous permeability.

BARRIER PROPERTIES OF SKIN

The skin's barrier properties reside essentially in the
stratum corneum layer of the epidermis since there is no
significant difference between these rate-limiting properties in isolated stratum corneum and full thickness epidermis (1). The absence of metabolic processes in the "dead"
keratinizing layers precludes any role for active transport
processes. Consequently, the stratum corneum acts as a
passive diffusion medium, but one which displays considerable diffusional resistance. The usual diffusion laws of
physics (Fick's law) apply to the phenomena of cutaneous
penetration, and steady penetration rates are proportional
to concentration differences across the membrane. The un-
derlying epidermal cell layers, the dermis, and the capil-
lary walls are relatively permeable. For a few substances
the dermal-epidermal basement membrane may constitute a
second barrier, but in general, once the stratum corneum is
traversed, penetration into the dermis and systemic circulation is assured.

In humans the skin surface is pierced by follicular orifices and sweat gland ducts. These provide alternate or
additional pathways for absorption, although the significance of sweat ducts in this process is questionable. For
substances penetrating the follicles, subsequent absorption
may occur through the follicular wall, sebaceous gland
duct, or sebaceous gland epithelium. The pilosebaceous
apparatus is an important route of entry for some substances and, in part, is more permeable than the interfol-
licular stratum corneum. For most substances both transepidermal and transappendageal routes play some role in absorption. Overall, however, the transepidermal route must
be the principal portal of entry for most materials, since
sweat gland ducts and hair follicle orifices account for
only 0.1-0.2% of the total skin surface area.

In the initial phase of percutaneous absorption after
topical application there may be transient but far greater
diffusion occurring through the transappendageal route than
through the transepidermal pathway (2). After steady-state
diffusion is attained (often within a few minutes) the dominant diffusion pathway is transepidermal rather than transappendageal. However, for certain large, slowly diffusing
molecules transappendageal penetration may be the predominant route throughout.

In regard to transepidermal absorption, the sites of
diffusional resistance in the stratum corneum layer reside
both in the plasma cell membrane and, predominantly, in the
poorly hydrated intracellular filament-matrix contents.
Substances traverse the stratum corneum directly through

keratinizing cells; the intercellular route must be of little
significance, presenting a volume of only about 1% of the
entire stratum corneum. Stratum corneum plasma cell membranes are structurally rigid and show remarkable chemical
resistance. These eembranes are about 150 Å thick, almost
double the 80 Å thickness found in basal cell plasma membranes. This change apparently results from surface deposition on, or inclusion of resistant material in or just beneath, stratum corneum plasma cell membranes (3), and this
may decrease cell permeability. Intracellularly, the keratin
matrix comprises about 65% of the cell mass, and the overall
water content is about 10%. For substances diffusing through
these cells keratin, lipids, and nonfibrous proteins constitute major "roadblocks" to passage. The keratin-matrix
structure is a mosaic of polar (bound water) and nonpolar
(interfilamentous lipid) regions which comprise parallel but
distinct diffusional pathways for water-soluble and lipid
molecules (2).

Overall, percutaneous absorption is a considerably more
complicated process than the prevailing passive diffusion
factors would suggest. The principal conditions affecting
cutaneous permeability are summarized in the remaining por-
tions of this paper.

PHYSICOCHEMICAL PROPERTIES OF PENETRANT

The solubility characteristics of a substance greatly influence its ability to penetrate the skin's barrier layer.
The classic Meyer-Overton theory of absorption claimed that
plasma cell membranes were constituted of mosaic patterns of
lipid and protein molecules: substances that were lipid
soluble penetrated the lipid portion of the membrane, while
water-soluble substances were absorbed after hydration of
proteins in the plasma cell membrane. In the case of the
stratum corneum barrier, however, significant diffusional resistance also arises within cells, once the plasma cell membranes have been crossed. Water-soluble compounds diffuse
through aqueous areas about the surface of keratin filaments,
while lipid-soluble substances pass through the interfilamentous lipids. Treherne (4) has roughly related the permeability constants of a series of compounds to their ether:
water partition coefficients and has stated that a partition
coefficient of unity favors percutaneous absorption. Nevertheless, the complex distribution of lipid and aqueous regions within stratum corneum cells often precludes accurate
predictions of permeability constants on the basis of ether:
water partition coefficients alone. Presumably, too, water
solubility assumes increased importance with increased hydration of the barrier layer.

Solubility of the penetrant within the vehicle is also a significant factor for percutaneous absorption. Greater solubility in the stratum corneum than in the vehicle increases surface concentrations and concentration gradients within the stratum corneum layer, promoting penetration. Some variation in penetration rates for solutes in different solvents has been demonstrated for several compounds, with water often enhancing absorption (5). Exogenous solvents are not a requirement for penetration to occur, however, as solids may be absorbed long after solvents volatilize. Despite penetrant-vehicle considerations, absorption rates are obviously modified further for substances that are bound to, or interact with, stratum corneum cells (salicylic acid, thioglycollic acid).

Electrolytes applied in aqueous solution usually do not penetrate well. Absorption of electrolytes occurs much more reasily through animal skin than through human skin, perhaps because pilosebaceous appendages, which have a much higher density per square millimeter in animals, play a significant role in absorption. Some ions of either sign will penetrate skin nearly as rapidly as water, but others are poorly absorbed (5). Ionization states are determined by pH and by the pK of the penetrant. Changes in the pH of a solution by 2 pH units on either side of the pK may induce ionization changes ranging from 0.1 to 99.9%. Artia (6) demonstrated that altering the pH of the skin to either side of neutrality caused increased skin permeability. Wedderburn showed that benzoic acid is 99.4% undissociated at pH 2 and only 1.6% undissociated at pH 6. Since it is the undissociated form that is absorbed, increased penetration occurs at pH 2 (7).

There is also a rough relationship between molecular size and percutaneous absorption, with the size of the penetrating molecule usually in inverse relationship to its rate of absorption. For example, human serum albumin passes through the barrier exceedingly slowly, in contrast to helium, which is quickly absorbed. While small molecules penetrate more rapidly than larger ones, within narrow ranges of molecular size there is little correlation between molecular size and rate of absorption. In general, molecules with molecular weights in excess of 3,000 penetrate poorly, but for some large molecules--even macromolecular compounds-- very slow absorption may occur. In certain homologous series of compounds, greater lipid solubility with increasing molecular weight may result in increasing penetration rates for the larger molecules. This effect has been shown in studies of homologous alcohols from methanol to octanol, for example (8).

Barrett et al. also found that a reduction in particle size increased the penetration of some drugs (9).

WATER

The skin's normal appearance, and its ability to resist environmental insults (irritants, toxins, etc.), largely derive from the stratum corneum's ability to bind water. Overall, normal corneal water content is about 10%, although a gradient from the innermost cells [approximating fully hydrated (80%) granular layer cells] to the outermost layer must exist.

An occlusive, impermeable covering over the skin greatly enhances the penetration of almost any substance placed on the skin surface by factors of 4 to 5 or more. This effect results from increased water retention in the stratum corneum layer, together with the increased skin surface temperature and, perhaps, blood flow, although prevention of mechanical removal of applied substances plays an auxiliary role. Prolonged application of occlusive dressings for 72 hr produces an excessively hydrated stratum corneum which develops multiple folds. Surface area estimations reveal a 37% increase over nonoccluded sites, suggesting that increased absorptive area, as well as increased water content, may facilitate penetration through hydrated stratum corneum (10). Nonetheless, even the highly hydrated horny layer still remains an effective barrier against penetration.

Measurements over a temperature range of 7°-49°C reveal that the amount of water absorbed or lost by human stratum corneum is influenced by temperature and relative humidity (11). When plotted on a semilogarithmic scale, water content of stratum corneum varies linearly with the relative humidity of the environment (11). Absolute humidity (moisture) is not a significant factor for water uptake. In regard to temperature effects, *in vitro* studies of human stratum corneum have shown that at relative humidity below 60% stratum corneum rapidly loses its ability to retain water with decreasing temperatures. Conversely, water content increases 50% when the temperature is raised from 20° to 35°C at relative humidity below 60% (12). Temperature dependence decreases with increasing relative humidity, until at 90% relative humidity no temperature dependence is demonstrable. Low temperatures in lower relative humidity ranges undoubtedly result in some loss of normal water content, reducing barrier pliability and producing corneal breaks, which lead to chapped or dry skin.

After immersion in water for a 3-day period, stratum corneum absorbs (or binds intracellularly) about six times its weight of water. Diffusion of water-soluble molecules through bound viscous water is much slower and more difficult than through straightforward aqueous solutions (13). The precise manner in which water is bound within corneal cells is unknown. Many years ago Szakall observed that water-soluble compounds within the barrier layer demonstrated strong hygroscopic properties, and that the content of these substances was markedly reduced in inflamed (psoriatic) skin sites (14). Singer and Vinson (11) later prepared stratum corneum extracts of low molecular weight, water-soluble substances which demonstrated marked avidity for water, and which they considered to be primarily responsible for water-binding in stratum corneum cells. Current theories concerning retention of cell water suggest that retained water is due to multilayer adsorption onto proteins. This phenomenon is at least partially dependent on certain "extended" protein conformations, where the backbone peptide groups polarize, orient, and retain deep layers of water (15). In stratum corneum cells, much water is probably bound in layers to intracellular keratin and, perhaps, other proteins, forming a water-rich polar region that widens interfibrillary spaces. Extension of these aqueous pathways undoubtedly facilitates percutaneous absorption after skin surface occlusion, which may increase barrier water content to 50% or more.

VEHICLES

Consideration of the effects of vehicles on percutaneous absorption are complex; only certain broad principles relating to this subject will be presented here.

Vehicles may significantly affect the penetration of substances through the horny layer (16), although experimental data regarding the "advantages" of one vehicle over another have often been conflicting (17). In general, the activity of the drug within the vehicle is more important than the properties of the vehicle itself. Unless an applied substance is capable of penetrating the barrier to some degree, the vehicle is of minor importance, provided that it does not damage stratum corneum cells and thereby enhance permeability.

The physical characteristics of the vehicle are a major consideration in its selection. Substances will be more rapidly released from vehicles having a low affinity for the penetrant. Pertinent factors here are related to the solubility of the penetrant in the vehicle, the rate of diffusion of the penetrant in the vehicle, and the rate of release of the penetrant from its base. Affinity of vehicular contents for incorporated substances reduces percutaneous absorption, as has been shown for propylene glycol gels containing adrenal steroids, for example (18).

Particle size, drug concentration in the vehicle, and, to some extent, viscosity of the vehicle are other significant factors. In the past some studies have attributed greater importance to vehicles in their effects on transappendageal, rather than on transepidermal, absorption, although added wetting agents were probably responsible for these observations (19).

The thermodynamic activity of the incorporated material is an important factor. Thermodynamic activity is the product of the concentration of the drug and its activity coefficient in the vehicle. Rapid release of the drug is dependent on its high thermodynamic activity in the vehicle, as the direction of flow is always from the higher to the lower thermodynamic potential (20). For specific concentrations of certain substances, it has been shown that thermodynamic activities may vary as much as 1,000-fold from one vehicle to another (20). Activity coefficients are reduced by such factors as pH differences (acidic compounds in alkaline vehicles) and complex formation with vehicular contents. Loosely held drugs have high activity coefficients; vehicles with relatively low solvent power for incorporated compounds will usually induce more rapid penetration (20). In general, a compound must be at least partially soluble in its vehicle so that it can be readily released into the receptor phase (skin barrier); high solubility may result in preferential retention in the vehicle. The rate of transfer of a compound from its base into the skin is related to the partition coefficient between the base and the barrier layer (stratum corneum-vehicle partition coefficient).

Drug concentration effects require brief comment. In general, concentration increases result in enhanced penetration, but--as for aliphatic alcohols--this is not always the case. Where increases do occur, they often are not directly proportional to drug concentrations but may increase more slowly, in proportion to the square root of concentration for some substances (21). For a few compounds (phenol, silver nitrate) higher concentrations produce caustic protein-precipitant effects, establishing a protective coat in the form of a crust which effectively reduces the penetration of any applied substance (22, 23).

The physical properties of vehicles are also important in the degree of occlusion they produce leading to water retention in the stratum corneum layer by reducing transepidermal water loss. The absorption-promoting effects of corneal hydration have been discussed above. Greases, oils, and collodion--the most occlusive vehicles--produce the greatest hydration of the barrier layer. For many substances, pharmacologic effects induced by increased absorption from these vehicles should be greater than from less occlusive bases such as powders, for example. Conversely, powders and glycerin-containing vehicles, especially under conditions of low relative humidity, may actually produce some dehydration of the stratum corneum layer and reduce permeability.

Not all vehicles are inert when applied to the skin surface. Certain nonaqueous bases promote penetration by producing structural or chemical damage in the barrier layer. Many of these vehicles are aprotic materials, accepting rather than donating protons: dimethyl sulfoxide (DMSO), dimethylacetamide, and dimethyl formamide are examples of these. The vehicles themselves also penetrate the barrier layer with ease.

The use of DMSO potentiates the percutaneous absorption of a wide variety of compounds, both organic and inorganic (24-27). Increases in penetration may be seen with DMSO concentrations as low as 15% (27), but highly significant increases often require concentrations of 60-80% or higher. For materials absorbed from the surface, 50% concentrations of DMSO also enhance the permeability of dermal connective tissue, apparently through the vehicle's depolymerizing effects on hyaluronic acid (28). Increased permeability of the barrier is reversed *in vivo* after aprotic solvent (DMSO) evaporation, but persistent damage has been found *in vitro*, presumably resulting from displacement of water and removal of lipids. Displacement of bound water by the solvent, partial extraction of lipids, and possible protein configurational changes resulting from replacement of water by the vehicle are responsible for enhanced passage of materials through corneal cells after application of aprotic solvents.

Refractive lens errors in laboratory animals were found after early investigations with DMSO. Initial enthusiasm for the topical use of DMSO has been further tempered by the frank irritation which may be produced by the relatively high concentrations required even in normal, let alone diseased, skin sites. Erythema, edema (especially perifollicular), burning, some itching, and unpleasant odor or taste may follow local application. In ultrastructural observations made some years ago with R. W. Pearson, we found that within 30 min after application of 75% DMSO to human skin there were vacuolar degenerative changes in epidermal cells and separation of the basement membrane from the basal cell layer.

Low molecular weight volatile solvents such as ether, methanol, ethanol, and acetone may also damage the skin's barrier layer. Substantial lipid extraction from stratum corneum cells, which leaves a more porous barrier, is most likely responsible for this effect.

SURFACTANTS

Ionic and nonionic surface active agents are widely used as emulsifiers and detergents in a number of household, cosmetic, and industrial preparations. Anionic and cationic surfactants damage the barrier layer of the skin even in concentrations as low as 1% (29). Acute histologic changes of epidermal cell degeneration, focal necrosis, and dermal inflammation may follow single or repeated applications of these compounds in laboratory animals; nonionic agents, however, have low irritant potential (30). Surfactants potentiate penetration: a 5% solution of sodium lauryl sulfate, for example, doubles the diffusion rate for water after 1 hr (31, 32). Surfactants are absorbed by the skin, though not readily; anionic substances pass through the barrier more easily than cationic or nonionic compounds. Laurate ion penetrates most effectively among anionic compounds and enhances absorption of other substances. There is also significant penetration by sodium salts of fatty acids with chain lengths of ten carbon atoms or less, though this process is dependent on variations in pH. Longer chain fatty acids are more poorly absorbed (33, 34).

Increased penetration induced by surfactants is largely due to protein (keratin) denaturation, a process which is accompanied by tissue swelling and which is at least partially reversible (35). The protein binding ability of surfactants is probably of primary significance both in the induction of epidermal cell damage by these compounds and in their alteration of barrier permeability. In addition, however, anionic surfactants also markedly reduce the amount of bound water in tissue (36); rehydration after removal of the surfactant partially restores barrier function. Reactions between surface active agents and plasma membrane lipids may well alter plasma membrane properties and also increase permeability. Surfactant reactions with collagen probably enhance *dermal* permeability as well.

SKIN SITE

The variations in permeability of skin in different body sites depend on the thickness of the intact stratum corneum and, to a lesser degree, the density of cutaneous appendages. Equally thick layers of stratum corneum from plantar skin and from the flexor surface of the forearm, for example, show equal penetrability (37).

Feldman and Maibach (38) used ^{14}C-labeled hydrocortisone to study differences in permeability in various anatomical regions of the body. Measuring [^{14}C]-steroid excretion in the urine, they found that the greatest total absorption of hydrocortisone occurred from the scrotum, with decreasing absorption from the forehead, scalp, back, forearms, palms, and plantar surface of the foot arch respectively. They concluded that for hydrocortisone permeability was greater in areas where pilosebaceous follicles were larger and more numerous, and the stratum corneum was thin. Penetrability was reduced where the barrier was thick, as on plantar surfaces. In other studies, however, it has been shown that for small molecules such as water, steady-state diffusion through plantar and palmar skin may exceed that of most other skin sites (2).

There is marked variability in the penetration rate when the same substance is applied to the same region of skin in different normal individuals. Marzulli (37) found that the absorption rate from the most permeable region (postauricular skin) in some individuals was comparable to the absorption rate from the least permeable region (plantar skin) in other normal individuals.

TEMPERATURE

Fluctuations in skin temperature will influence the absorption of topical agents. Under normal *in vivo* conditions the range of skin surface temperatures is obviously quite limited. Nevertheless, for several compounds temperature coefficients of 1.4-3 have been found in temperature ranges of 20°-40°C (5). In one study, for example, the temperature of excised human skin was increased from 10° to 40°C, while the relative humidity was maintained at 50%; penetration of [^{14}C]-acetylsalicylic acid was found to increase almost 15-fold by increasing the skin temperature only (38).

For lipid-soluble substances at least, lowered viscosity of tissue lipids at higher temperatures reduces activation energies for diffusion. For certain materials which penetrate skin rapidly (inert gases, for example) the enhancing effects of raised temperatures result chiefly from progressive vasodilatation.

In clinical dermatologic practice the use of occlusive plastic film wrappings produces skin surface temperature increases which potentiate penetration. Although substances applied under occlusion are absorbed much more readily, this effect is importantly augmented by the subsequent hydration of the stratum corneum.

PERIPHERAL CIRCULATION

The peripheral circulation, or blood flow through the dermis, has some effect on percutaneous absorption since it helps to determine the concentration gradients of topically applied compounds and the length of time the penetrant will

remain in the skin. In perfused dog skin preparations some
effects on penetration of tri-*n*-butyl phosphate were shown
after both increased and decreased rates of perfusate flow
(39). *In vivo* this effect of circulatory flow in tissue
largely concerns the penetration of rapidly absorbed compounds such as gases and small lipid-soluble molecules. For
most other substances percutaneous absorption is limited by
the stratum corneum layer.

To some degree hyperemia increases the absorption of the
penetrant by increasing concentration gradients between the
skin surface and dermis. This effect can be shown dramatically for certain gases which penetrate normal skin readily,
when carbon dioxide is used to induce vasodilatation (40).
Conversely, where vasoconstriction was induced by topical
methylprednisolone applied to damaged (stripped) skin sites,
subsequent absorption of topical testosterone-4-^{14}C was significantly reduced (41). However, often when hyperemia is
present, as in damaged or inflamed skin sites, concomitant
alterations in barrier integrity may be the major factor promoting increased absorption of the penetrant.

THE DERMAL-EPIDERMAL JUNCTION

After penetration of the entire epidermis, further passage
of absorbed materials into the corium and then into the systemic circulation is usually assured. For some substances,
however, there appears to be a second barrier at the dermal-
epidermal junction. Presumably the site of this barrier co-
incides with the basement membrane, a collagen-like structure
said to consist of scleroprotein, glycoprotein, and mucopoly-
saccharide protein. Many years ago it was demonstrated that
when thorium X solutions (thorium chloride) were applied to
human skin, autoradiographs showed diffusion of thorium X
throughout the epidermis but with negligible passage of material into the corium (42, 43). After iontophoresis, however,
thorium X could be readily demonstrated in the corium (44).
Similar roughly qualitative differences in electrolyte penetration of epidermis versus dermis were shown for ^{32}P-labeled
sodium phosphate (45). In general, permeability of full
thickness human skin for ions is poor, presumably because the
hydration sphere about the ion yields a relatively large diffusing particle (compared to water) and because the ionic
charge is capable of reacting with other tissue charges.
Diffusion through appendages may play a relatively larger
role for electrolytes, as autoradiography in these studies
suggested.

Later investigations of basement membrane barrier effects,
however, revealed ready passage of inorganic phosphorus and

chloride ions *in vitro* (46). In similar studies methylene blue and Evans blue failed to pass through the dermal-epidermal junction, but readily penetrated when the basement membrane was removed (46). Basement membrane penetrability was enhanced by exposure to hyaluronidase or to collagenase (46). Recently, it was suggested that urea or lactamide might be clinically useful in increasing basement membrane permeability (47).

SPECIES VARIATIONS

Skin is significantly less permeable in humans than it is in other mammals. Presumably differences in stratum corneum thickness and, perhaps, structure, as well as in density of pilosebaceous appendages per unit area, are largely responsible for this finding. While relationships between species are not consistent for different substances, the general permeability order is rabbit > rat > guinea pig or pig > humans (5). The most striking species differences are seen for electrolytes.

AGE

The relationship between age and percutaneous absorption has received inadequate attention, particularly in regard to skin permeability in aged individuals. Normal or inflamed skin sites in infants *appear* to be more permeable than in adults, as attested by reports of Cushingoid side-effects complicating topical use of certain adrenal steroids. Detailed quantitative absorption data in infants and children have not yet been reported.

BARRIER INTEGRITY

As might be expected, mechanical trauma sufficient to produce interruptions in barrier continuity increases that layer's permeability. While physical absence of the barrier is largely responsible for this effect, some of the increased permeability results from the ensuing vasodilatation, which enhances skin surface to dermis diffusion gradients.

When the barrier is removed with adhesive cellophane tape, evaporative loss of water from the skin is roughly equivalent to that from a free water surface. If large areas of the body were denuded of the barrier layer, water loss would reach 2 l daily (48). Studies of hydrocortisone-4-^{14}C (41), testosterone-4-^{14}C (41), phenol (48), and a wide variety of other compounds have demonstrated marked increases --up to several hundred-fold--in percutaneous absorption after damage to or removal of the stratum corneum layer. Even under these circumstances, however, penetration rates through the remaining epidermal cell layers vary considerably for different compounds, as has been shown for cortisone-4-^{14}C and hydrocortisone-4-^{14}C, for example (49). Presumably these differences in penetration rates reflect variations in ether: water partition coefficients, since it appears that the living cell layers of the epidermis are more significant barriers to the absorption of nonpolar than polar molecules.

Some direct or indirect enhancement of percutaneous absorption has also been claimed for the effects of ultraviolet light, ionizing radiation, red and short-wave infrared rays, and mild thermal burns (see Ref. 50). Some of these claims have not been well substantiated or confirmed, however. A variety of chemical agents--mustard gas, alkalies, acids, etc.--also injure barrier cells and increase permeability.

Irritation or endogenous inflammation of the skin, resulting in altered keratinization, is also associated with increased permeability. Penetration of testosterone-4-^{14}C is 2 1/2 to 4 times greater through psoriatic patches than through normal skin sites, for example (50). Comparisons of pyribenzamine absorption from a 10% cream applied to normal and to psoriatic skin sites revealed that 12 hr later significant excretion of drug in urine occurred only in psoriatic patients (51). Similarly enhanced penetration of a variety of compounds has been found in patients with seborrheic dermatitis, exfoliative dermatitis, atopic dermatitis, and other inflammatory skin disorders.

After injury or removal, barrier function in humans returns almost to normal within 3 days (41). This temporary barrier is composed of parakeratotic cells and persists until the regenerating epidermis is capable of forming normally keratinizing cells. Usually these parakeratotic cells are sloughed between 6 and 11 days after stripping (52). Complete regeneration of the stratum corneum requires approximately 2 weeks, at which time functional integrity is entirely restored.

DRUG BINDING AND METABOLISM

In the past, many studies have been devoted to the elucidation of physical and chemical data pertinent to basic mechanisms of percutaneous absorption. Much information has also been accumulated on the quantitative absorption of a large number of compounds. The question of what happens to a given substance once it has penetrated the barrier layer

has received much less attention. The subjects of local pharmacokinetics, protein binding, tissue storage, skin cell receptor sites (for sex hormones, glucocorticoids, etc.), and
the metabolism and interaction of absorbed drugs or toxins
require much more extensive investigation.

In recent years sensitive and reliable techniques have
been developed for the measurement of drug concentrations and
for detection of drugs and metabolites in body fluids and
tissues. With the broad exceptions of carcinogens and
steroid compounds (53, 54), these techniques for metabolic
studies have not yet been extensively explored or utilized in
the skin. The subjects of optimal size and frequency of individual "doses" (local applications) and rates of tissue
accumulation and elimination also require further study.
Presumably, the distribution half-life of compounds in epidermis and dermis is much shorter than their elimination half-
life and their rate of absorption is proportional both to
tissue concentration and to rate of metabolism and/or elimination. The question of whether drug half-lives in tissue become longer with larger doses, as might be expected, needs
further investigation.

Accumulation of compounds stored in the skin may occur,
especially with repeated administration. In studies we performed some years ago with ^{14}C-labeled triamcinolone acetonide
applied once to "stripped" skin sites for 8 hr, some retained
steroid was still present in application site biopsies 36 hr
later. For some compounds, connective tissue or subcutaneous
fat may represent important depot sites. Solubility or binding characteristics of a substance, especially for fat or
protein, occurring naturally or deliberately induced by
molecular manipulation, may significantly enhance or prolong
pharmacologic effects. Whether storage or metabolism of absorbed compounds is significantly different in normal versus
inflamed skin sites has not been systematically studied.

Biotransformation of absorbed compounds in skin or appendages usually results in the production of inactive metabolites, but occasionally metabolically active compounds are
formed. The conversion of cortisone to hydrocortisone (53)
and testosterone to dihydrotestosterone in skin or appendages
(54) are examples of the latter. The pharmacologic activity
of a substance transformed into active matabolites obviously
cannot be predicted from the parent compound's pharmacokinetics alone. Enzymatic metabolic pathways in skin (oxidative,
reductive, hydrolytic, etc.), possible conjugation reactions,
and other factors affecting cutaneous metabolism of absorbed
substances (age, skin disease or injury, etc.), are important
subjects for future investigation. The effects of enzyme induction and consequent metabolic transformation induced by a
second compound, administered locally or taken systemically,

are unexplored.

Many compounds absorbed through the skin must be bound in part to tissue proteins or perhaps, in inflamed sites, to serum albumin (55) diffusing into the dermis through more permeable blood vessel walls. Bound compounds are presumably inactive, protected from biotransformation, and little able to diffuse out of the skin into blood vessel lumina. Since binding is usually reversible, the protein-drug complex serves as a local tissue reservoir, releasing drug as the free compound is removed via the circulation. The extent of possible protein binding and the specific proteins bound by compounds absorbed into the skin are largely unknown. The effect of a second compound with high protein affinity, locally applied or systemically administered, on both the binding and pharmacologic activity of the first substance can only be speculated upon. Age factors may influence protein binding, being lower in the very young and old, as shown for serum albumin (56, 57). Temperature, pH, and ionic strength can also affect the number of protein binding sites and their dissociation constants (58, 59). Marked differences among compounds in the extent of their binding to protein are only partially explicable; actively bound drugs usually have an ionizable acidic group at physiologic pH, are often double-ringed molecules, and are hydrophobic. Drug metabolites are usually less hydrophobic and are less actively bound to proteins than the parent compound. The effects of local disease states in skin on the concentration or binding properties of tissue proteins are purely a matter for speculation at the present time.

REFERENCES

1. Berenson, P. S., and Burch, G. E. (1971). Studies of diffusion through dead human skin. *Am. J. Trop. Med. Hyg. 31*:842.
2. Scheuplein, R. J., and Blank, I. H. (1971). Permeability of the skin. *Physiol. Rev. 51*:702.
3. Matoltsy, A. G., and Parakkal, P. F. (1965). Membrane-coating granules of keratinizing epithelia. *J. Cell. Biol. 24*:297.
4. Treherne, J. E. (1956). Permeability of skin to some non-electrolytes. *J. Physiol. 133*:171.
5. Tregear, R. T. (1966). *Physical Functions of Skin.* New York, Academic Press.
6. Artia, T., Hori, R., Anmo, T., Washitake, M., Akatsu, M., Yajima, T. (1970). Studies on percutaneous absorption of drugs. I. *Chem. Pharm. Bull. Tokyo 18*:1045.

7. Wedderburn, D. L. (1964). *Advances in Pharmaceutical Sciences,* Vol. I., p. 195. New York, Academic Press.

8. Blank, I. H., and Scheuplein, R. J. (1964). Design of topical drug products: Biopharmaceutics. In *Progress in the Biological Sciences in Relation to Dermatology,* eds. A. Rook and R. H. Champion, Vol. 2, p. 164. Cambridge University Press, Cambridge.

9. Barrett, C. W., Hadgraft, J. W., and Sarkany, I. (1964). The influence of vehicles on skin penetration. *J. Pharm. Pharmacol. 16*:Suppl. 104T.

10. Harris, D. R., Papa, C. M., and Stanton, R. (1974). Percutaneous absorption and the surface area of occluded skin. *Br. J. Dermatol. 91*:27.

11. Singer, E. J., and Vinson, L. J. (1966). The water-binding properties of skin. *Proc. Sci. Sect. Toilet Goods Assoc. 46*:29.

12. Spencer, T. S., Linamen, C. E., and Jones, H. E. (1975). Temperature dependence of water content of stratum corneum. *Br. J. Dermatol. 93*:159.

13. Scheuplein, R. J., and Morgan, L. J. (1967). "Bound-water" in keratin membranes measured by a microbalance technique. *Nature 214*:456.

14. Szakall, A. (1955). Über die Eigenschaften, Herkunft und physiologischen Funktionen der die H-tonenkonzentration bestimmendun Wirkstoffe in der verhornten Epidermis. *Arch. Klin. Dermatol. 201*:331.

15. Ling, G. W., and Walton, C. L. (1976). What retains water in living cells? *Science 191*:293.

16. Poulsen, B. J. (1973). In *Drug Design,* ed. E. J. Ariens, p. 349. New York, Academic Press.

17. Malkinson, F. D., and Rothman, S. (1961). Percutaneous absorption. In *Handbuch der Haut und Geschlechtskrankheiten,* Vol. 1, Part III. eds. A. Marchionini and H. W. Spier. Berlin, Springer, Verlag.

18. Poulsen, B. J., Young, E., Coquilla, V., and Katz, M. (1968). The effect of topical vehicle composition on the *in vitro* release of fluocinolone acetonide and its acetate ester. *J. Pharm. Sci. 57*:928.

19. Mackee, G. M., Sulzberger, M. B., Herrmann, F., and Baer, R. L. (1945). Histologic studies on percutaneous penetration, with special reference to the effect of vehicles. *J. Invest. Dermatol. 6*:43.

20. Higuchi, T. (1960). Physical chemical analysis of percutaneous absorption process from creams and ointments. *J. Soc. Cosmet. Chem. 11*:85.

21. Hlynka, J. N., Anderson, A. J., and Riedel, B. E. (1969). Investigations of intracutaneous drug absorption. II. A comparison of intracutaneous and systemic absorption as functions of rest time and concentration. *Can. J. Pharm. Sci. 4*:92.

22. Macht, D. I. (1938). The absorption of drugs and poisons through the skin and mucous membranes. *J. Am. Med. Assoc.* *110*:409.

23. Nørgaard, O. (1954). Investigations with radioactive Ag[111] into the resorption of silver through human skin. *Acta Derm.-Venereol.* *35*:415.

24. Stoughton, R. B., and Fritsch, W. C. (1964). Influence of dimethyl sulfoxide on human percutaneous absorption. *Arch. Dermatol.* *90*:512.

25. Kligman, A. M. (1965). Topical pharmacology and toxicology of dimethyl sulfoxide. Part I. *J. Am. Med. Assoc.* *193*:796.

26. Sweeney, T. M., Downes, A. M., and Matoltsy, A. G. (1966). The effect of dimethyl sulfoxide on the epidermal water barrier. *J. Invest. Dermatol.* *46*:300.

27. Stelzer, J. M., Jr., Colaizzi, J. L., and Wurdack, P. J. (1968). Influence of dimethylsulfoxide on percutaneous absorption of salicylic acid and sodium salicylate from ointments. *J. Pharm. Sci.* *57*:1732.

28. Fabianek, J., and Herp, A. (1966). Studies of the effect of dimethylsulfoxide on permeability of dermal connective tissue. *Proc. Soc. Exp. Biol. Med.* *122*:290.

29. Malten, K. E., Spruit, D., Bolmaars, H. G. M., and de Keizer, M. J. M. (1968). Horny layer injury by solvents. *Berufsdermatosen* *16*:135.

30. Lansdown, A. B. H., and Grasso, P. (1972). Physicochemical factors influencing epidermal damage by surface active agents. *Br. J. Dermatol.* *86*:361.

31. Sprott, W. E. (1965). Surfactants and percutaneous absorption. *Trans. St. John's Hosp. Dermatol. Soc.* *51*:186.

32. Baker, H. J., and Kligman, A. M. (1967). Measurement of transepidermal water loss by electrical hygrometry. *Arch. Dermatol.* *96*:441.

33. Blank, I. H., and Gould, E. (1959). Penetration of anionic surfactants (surface active agents) into skin: I. Penetration of sodium laurate and sodium dodecyl sulfate into excised human skin. *J. Invest. Dermatol.* *33*:327.

34. Blank, I. H., and Gould, E. (1961). Penetration of anionic surfactants into skin. II. Study of mechanisms which impede the penetration of synthetic anionic surfactants into skin. *J. Invest. Dermatol.* *37*:311.

35. Scheuplein, R. J., and Ross, L. (1970). Effect of surfactants on the permeability of the epidermis. *J. Soc. Cosmet. Chem.* *21*:853.

36. Blank, I. H., and Shappirio, E. B. (1955). The water content of the stratum corneum. III. Effect of previous contact with aqueous solutions of soaps and detergents. *J. Invest. Dermatol.* *25*:391.

37.   Marzulli, F. N. (1962). Barriers to skin penetration. *J. Invest. Dermatol. 39*:387.

38.   Feldman, R. J., and Maibach, H. I. (1967). Regional variation in percutaneous penetration of ^{14}C-cortisol in man. *J. Invest. Dermatol. 48*:181.

39.   Kjaersgaard, A. R. (1954). Perfusion of isolated dog skin, using the saphenous artery. *J. Invest. Dermatol. 22*:135.

40.   McClellan, W. S., and Comstock, C. (1949). The cutaneous absorption of radon from naturally carbonated water baths. *Arch. Phys. Med. 30*:29.

41.   Malkinson, F. D. (1958). Studies on the percutaneous absorption of C^{14} labeled steroids by use of the gas-flow cell. *J. Invest. Dermatol. 31*:19.

42.   Witten, V. H., Ross, M. S., Oshry, E., and Hyman, A. B. (1951). Studies of thorium X applied to human skin. I. Routes and degree of penetration and sites of deposition of thorium X applied in selected vehicles. *J. Invest. Dermatol. 17*:311.

43.   Witten, V. H., Ross, M. S., Oshry, E., and Holstrom, V. (1953). Studies of thorium X applied to human skin. II. Comparative findings of the penetration and localization of thorium X when applied in alcoholic solution, in ointment, and in lacquer vehicles. *J. Invest. Dermatol. 20*:93.

44.   Fleischmajer, R., and Witten, V. H. (1955). Studies of thorium X applied to human skin. IV. Clinical and autoradiographic findings following the introduction by iontophoresis. *J. Invest. Dermatol. 25*:223.

45.   Witten, V. H., Brauer, E. W., Loevinger, R., and Holmstrom, V. (1956). Studies of radioactive phosphorus (P^{32}) applied to human skin. I. Erythema and autoradiographic findings following application in various forms. *J. Invest. Dermatol. 26*:437.

46.   Ohkubo, T., and Sano, S. (1973). Functional aspects of dermo-epidermal junction. *Acta. Dermatovzer. (Stockholm) Suppl. 73*:121.

47.   Handschumacher, R. E. (1974). Aspects of pharmacology pertinent to the skin. *Clin. Pharmacol. Ther. 16*:865.

48.   Monash, S., and Blank, H. (1958). Location and reformation of the epithelial barrier to water vapor. *Arch. Dermatol. 78*:710.

49.   Malkinson, F. D. (1962). Radioactive agents and radio-isotopes in dermatology. Investigative applications. *12th Int. Congr. Dermatol. 1*:657.

50.   Malkinson, F. D. (1964). Permeability of the stratum corneum. In *The Epidermis*, eds. W. Montagna and W. C. Lobitz, Jr., p. 435. New York, Academic Press.

51. Michelfelder, T. T., and Peck, S. M. (1952). Absorption of pyribenzamine through intact and damaged skin. *J. Invest. Dermatol. 19*:237.

52. Spruit, D., and Malten, K. E. (1965). Epidermal water-barrier formation after stripping of normal skin. *J. Invest. Dermatol. 45*:6.

53. Malkinson, F. D., Lee, M. W., and Cutukovich, I. (1959). *In vitro* studies of adrenal steroid metabolism in the skin. *J. Invest. Dermatol. 32*:101.

54. Gomez, E. C., and Hsia, S. L. (1968). *In vitro* metabolism of testosterone-4-^{14}C and $^{4}\Delta$-androstene-3, 17-dione-4^{14}C in human skin. *Biochemistry 7*:24.

55. Goldstein, A., Kalman, S. M., and Aronow, L. (1969). *Principles of Drug Action*, pp. 106-205. New York, Harper and Row.

56. Krasner, J., Giacoia, G. P., and Yaffe, S. J. (1973). Drug-protein binding in the newborn infant. *Ann. N.Y. Acad. Sci. 226*:101.

57. Hooper, W. D., Bochner, F., Eadie, M. J., and Tyrer, J. H. (1974). Plasma protein binding of diphenylhydantoin: Effects of sex hormones, renal and hepatic disease. *Clin. Pharmacol. Ther. 15*:276.

58. Lunde, P. K. M., Rane, A., Yaffe, S. J., Lund, L., and Sjoqvest, F. (1970). Plasma protein binding of diphenylhydantoin in man: Interaction with other drugs and the effect of temperature and plasma dilution. *Clin. Pharmacol. Ther. 11*:846.

59. Sellers, E. M., and Koch-Weser, J. (1974). Binding of diazoxide and other benzothiadiazines to human albumin. *Biochem. Pharmacol. 23*:553.

New Procedures for Evaluating Cutaneous Absorption

Jane E. Shaw, S. K. Chandrasekaran,
Patricia S. Campbell, and Leonore G. Schmitt

Research Laboratories
ALZA Corporation
Palo Alto, California

We are developing a new class of dosage forms called
therapeutic systems which are defined both by their rate and
duration of drug delivery. Transdermal therapeutic systems
are designed to control delivery of drug to the surface of
intact skin, at rates well below the maximum the skin can
accept; drug then diffuses through the epidermis, and passes
via the capillaries to the general circulation. Control over
the rate at which drug permeates skin and enters the circulation resides, therefore, in the design of the transdermal
therapeutic system.

To design the optimum profile for release of drug from
such a therapeutic system, it is necessary to: (i) identify
the pattern of drug input to the systemic circulation which
will elicit the required pharmacological response, while mini-
mizing unwanted pharmacological effects, and (ii) determine
whether the drug will permeate skin in the required therapeutic amount. To evaluate the latter it is necessary to gain
an understanding of the mechanisms which influence permeation
and immobilization of drugs in intact skin.

We have developed an *in vitro* test, which utilizes
cadaver skin mounted as a membrane in a diffusion chamber, to
follow the permeation and immobilization of drugs in human
skin. The results obtained have been predictive of cutaneous
absorption and transdermal permeation *in vivo* (1).

The first transdermal therapeutic system to be studied

clinically delivers the drug scopolamine at the rate that pre-
vents motion-induced nausea, but avoids, in all but a small
minority of subjects, other parasympatholytic effects of the
drug. The system functions for 3 days.

     An understanding of the factors which influence cutaneous
and percutaneous absorption, together with advances in polymer technology, have led to the possibility of providing optimal drug therapy for the treatment of systemic disorders--
acute or chronic--by means of controlled, unattended administration of a drug to the skin surface, for prolonged, predetermined periods of time.

IN VITRO SKIN PERMEATION STUDIES

     The permeation of drugs through human skin *in vitro* was
determined as previously described (1, 2). Samples, from
human cadavers, of whole skin, epidermis, or dermis were
mounted as membranes in diffusion chambers, and solutions
containing radiolabeled drug were placed in contact with one
surface. The permeation of drug was then followed at 30°C.

Effect of Concentration and pH on Permeation of Scopolamine

     Aqueous solutions of [^{3}H] scopolamine of different concen-
trations and pH were placed in contact with the stratum corneum surface of intact skin. The values obtained for the
steady-state flux of scopolamine (in µg/cm^2/hr) are illustrated in Figure 1. We determined that transdermal flux

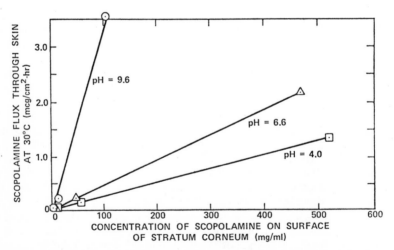

Fig. 1. *Effect of concentration and pH on scopolamine flux
through human skin* in vitro.

increases either with increasing concentration or with increasing pH. For scopolamine, as a result of increasing the
pH of the donor solution from 4 to 9, the drug is converted
primarily from the salt to its base form. The more lipophilic
base form is the more rapidly permeating form of the drug.

Permeation through Epidermis and Dermis

Further *in vitro* studies indicated that permeation of
scopolamine free base from saturated aqueous solutions through
whole skin occurs at a rate similar to the rate of permeation
through epidermis alone. In contrast, permeation through the
dermis is greater than through either whole skin or epidermis
by more than two orders of magnitude. These data, shown in
Table 1, indicate that the epidermis offers the major resistance to transdermal permeation of scopolamine through

TABLE 1

Permeation Behavior of Scopolamine from Saturated Aqueous
Solutions

Drug Form	Skin	Skin thickness, mils	Steady-state flux, $\mu g/cm^2/hr$
Free base	Whole skin	37.5	6.0
	Epidermis	2.0	6.7
	Dermis	35.0	1342
Salt	Whole skin	37.5	0.8
	Dermis	35.0	5710

intact skin. Permeation of scopolamine hydrobromide from
aqueous solutions through whole skin occurred at lower rates
than permeation of scopolamine base, but through the dermis
alone, permeation of scopolamine hydrobromide occurred at
higher rates than the base. The latter phenomenon is probably associated with the increased water solubility of the
salt form of the drug.

Permeation through Skin Obtained from Different Areas

The permeation of scopolamine base from aqueous solution through the rate-limiting epidermis *in vitro* was found to vary, depending upon the site from which the skin was excised. The steady-state flux of scopolamine, when using donor solutions of two different concentrations placed in contact with the stratum corneum surface of skin obtained from the thigh and postauricular area of the same cadaver, is listed in Table 2. For each concentration of drug tested, the greater steady-state flux was observed through skin from the postauricular area.

Upon completion of each permeation experiment the tissue was removed from the perfusion chamber, digested, and an aliquot counted, in order to determine the scopolamine content of the tissue, at the time when the steady-state permeation of scopolamine had been established. In this experiment it was demonstrated that the scopolamine content was lowest in epidermis from the postauricular area (Table 3). Since epidermal thickness varies in these two regions, the scopolamine content of the tissue has been expressed as quantity of drug per unit volume of skin (mg/ml).

Mathematical Model of Factors Controlling Drug Permeation

Based upon the results of such *in vitro* studies, we have developed a mathematical model of the drug permeation process which describes the penetration of micromolecular drugs through skin as a process of dissolution and diffusion. In this model, the transdermal flux of drug is depicted as being through a composite multilayer membrane, with the stratum corneum modeled as a heterogeneous membrane of lipid interspersed with protein. The model allows one to correlate drug flux with the water and oil solubilities of the drug. We find that drug permeation through skin is predictable with this model (2, 3).

DEVELOPMENT OF A TRANSDERMAL THERAPEUTIC SYSTEM

An understanding of some of the factors which influence transdermal permeation of scopolamine *in vitro* allowed the development of a transdermal therapeutic system for scopolamine; systems were designed to deliver the drug at various rates to the surface of the skin, and hence to the systemic circulation. The different rates of continuous scopolamine delivery were evaluated for their ability to prevent nausea and vomiting due to motion.

TABLE 2

Permeation and Immobilization of Scopolamine in Epidermis

Skin	Scopolamine in donor, mg/ml	Epidermal thickness, cm	Scopolamine in epidermis, mg/ml	Scopolamine steady-state flux, μg/cm² /hr
Thigh	4.6 16.9	.0106	16.9 25.7	4.7 15.5
Postauricular	4.6 16.9	.0084	7.4 13.9	10.0 24.3

TABLE 3

Scopolamine and Protein Content of Stratum Corneum from Back and Postauricular Area, after 48 hr Wearing of Transdermal Therapeutic System-scopolamine

| Subject | Site stripped under TTS-Scopolamine | Total Stripping | | Stripping containing measurable amounts of scopolamine[a] | | |
		Number to glistening layer	Protein content, μg	Number	Protein content, μg	Scopolamine content, μg
482	Back	20	356	10	198	72.7
	Postauricular	22	328	10	181	44.0
481	Back	22	412	12	303	48.4
	Postauricular	25	405	8	185	15.5

[a] Limit of scopolamine assay was ~0.5 μg per stripping.

88

The result of this testing program is the Transdermal Therapeutic System-scopolamine (TTS-scopolamine), shown schematically in Figure 2. The system is a multilayer laminate, comprised of a drug reservoir containing scopolamine in a gel, sandwiched between an impermeable backing membrane and a rate-controlling microporous membrane. On the cutaneous side of the rate-controlling membrane is an adhesive gel, containing scopolamine; this gel layer serves both as an adhesive to secure the system on the skin surface and as a reservoir for a priming dose of drug to provide an initial quantity of drug prior to the establishment of controlled delivery of drug to the skin surface.

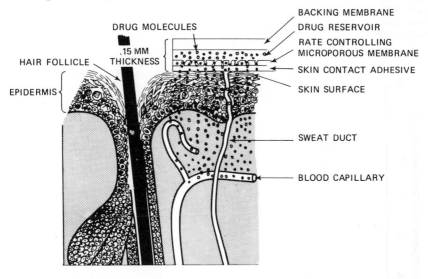

Fig. 2. Schematic illustration of Transdermal Therapeutic System-scopolamine in place on surface of intact skin. This system (1.6 cm^2 area) delivered 6 μg scopolamine base per hour.

The transport characteristics of scopolamine from the system are determined by molecular diffusion through the various elements of the multilayer laminate. During the priming dose period, drug diffusion from the contact adhesive layer dominates the temporal pattern of drug release. However, during steady-state delivery, rate-limitation or control is provided by the microporous membrane; this element ensures that the rate of delivery of scopolamine to the surface of the skin is less than the rate at which skin can absorb the drug, and hence the system, and not the skin, controls the entry of drug into the systemic circulation.

IN VIVO VERSUS IN VITRO FUNCTIONALITY OF THE SYSTEM

The release of scopolamine over a 24 hr period from a TTS-scopolamine *in vitro* is illustrated in Figure 3. To follow the rate of drug input to the systemic circulation during topical application of a TTS-scopolamine, we monitored the rate of urinary excretion of the drug, using a sensitive and specific assay (4). Taking into account the fact that following intramuscular or intravenous administration of scopolamine only 10% of the drug is recovered in the urine in the free

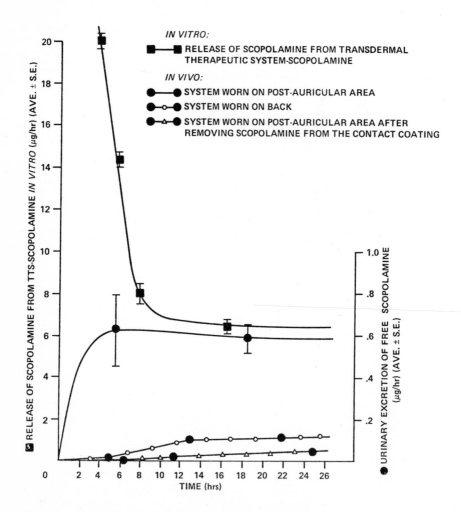

Fig. 3. Functionality of TTS-scopolamine in vitro *and in* vivo. *Urinary excretion of free scopolamine = 9.5 ± 0.9% (ave. + S.E.) of total drug administered.*

form, we observe that within approximately 4 hr following application of the system the rate of drug excretion approaches the predicted value of 0.1 times the rate of drug release from the system *in vitro.**   Approximately 18 hr later the same relation exists. Thus, the *in vivo* and *in vitro* release of drug from the TTS-scopolamine are similar.

The provision of a priming dose of drug serves to saturate the immobilization sites for scopolamine within the skin and hence permits rapid establishment of steady-state plasma levels, and urinary excretion of the drug; removal of this priming dose of drug from the contact adhesive reduces the drug input to the systemic circulation, for when the drug is released at a low constant rate it takes many hours to achieve saturation of the immobilization sites for the drug within the skin (Figure 3).

When the TTS-scopolamine is placed on other sites (e.g., the back) less permeable than the postauricular area, the less permeable skin cannot accept the drug at the rate provided by the system. In this situation the skin, and not the system, controls the input of scopolamine to the systemic circulation. Hence the amount of drug reaching the circulation is reduced (Figure 3).

REGIONAL DIFFERENCES IN SKIN PROPERTIES *IN VIVO*

Further examination of the regional differences in skin absorption *in vivo* were conducted by successively placing TTS-scopolamine (80 µg priming dose, 1.2 µg/hr for 48 hr) on the back and postauricular area of each of two subjects.

The urinary excretion of free drug during wearing of TTS-scopolamine is illustrated in Figure 4. For each subject the postauricular area was more permeable, as manifested by the greater rate of drug excretion. Following application of the system to the postauricular area of Subject 482, the rate of scopolamine excretion rose gradually and then remained constant at a level of approximately 0.1 µg/hr during wearing of the system. When the system was worn on the back of the same subject the skin offered resistance to drug input, since the rate of drug excretion *in vivo* did not approach the predicted value for steady-state urinary excretion of 0.12 µg/hr (10% of the 1.2 µg/hr released *in vitro*). When wearing the system on the back, Subject 481, within a few hours of application of the system, excreted drug at a rate which indicated that the system was controlling the rate of drug input

---

*Following intramuscular and intravenous administration of scopolamine only 10% of the drug was recovered in the urine as unchanged drug.

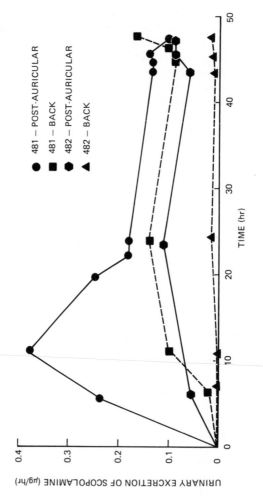

Fig. 4. Urinary excretion of free scopolamine during 48 hr wearing of Transdermal Therapeutic System-scopolamine.

92

to the circulation. When wearing the system on the post-auricular area, this subject had a high rate of drug excretion during the hours following application of the system. The possibility that this may result from decreased immobilization of drug within the epidermis of this subject, and hence increased drug input to the systemic circulation during that time when the priming dose of drug is delivered from the system, was confirmed by stripping the skin beneath the TTS-scopolamine with Scotch brand cellophane tape to glistening, and determining the protein and scopolamine content of successive strippings (Table 3).

For the two subjects both the protein and scopolamine content within skin strippings from the back were higher than those in strippings from the post auricular area. The scopolamine content of both skin sites from Subject 481 was less than that for equivalent areas from Subject 482, indicating individual differences in skin properties. For both subjects the highest rate of urinary excretion of scopolamine base was associated with least immobilization of drug within the stratum corneum.

TRANSDERMAL THERAPEUTIC SYSTEM-SCOPOLAMINE

The TTS-scopolamine, developed for application to the postauricular area for prevention of motion-induced nausea, is designed to minimize the observed differences in skin properties between individuals. The rate of steady-state release of drug is designed to be a fraction of the rate which the least permeable skin will accept, and the priming dose is designed such that all subjects attain a therapeutic level of drug within an acceptable time period following application of the system. The system is 2.5 cm^2 in area and its strength is specified by its temporal pattern of drug release: 200 µg priming dose, 10 µg/hr for 72 hr. For those subjects whose skin immobilizes less scopolamine we have determined that the higher rate of drug input to the systemic circulation during the first few hours following application of the system elicits no untoward pharmacological effect.

Results of large scale clinical studies have indicated that the TTS-scopolamine is a safe and effective dosage form for systemic administration of scopolamine for prevention of motion-induced nausea (5). The pattern of systemic delivery of scopolamine from the TTS-scopolamine permits realization of the antiemetic activity of the drug, with minimal incidence of other troublesome parasympatholytic effects of scopolamine, which are inescapable with conventional dosage forms.

CONCLUSIONS

To date, methods utilized to quantify the percutaneous absorption of drugs have been based on the amount of radioactivity excreted following application of a known amount of labeled compound to the skin surface. To correct for retention of radioactivity and excretion via other routes, urinary excretion data obtained after topical administration of a drug have been compared with the data obtained following intravenous administration of the same drug (6).

Using human skin *in vitro*, we have defined some of the factors which can modify not only the permeation but also immobilization of drugs in skin tissue; such factors include the concentration of drug applied to the skin surface, the physicochemical form of the drug, and the region of the body from which the skin sample is obtained. An insight into some of the factors which control percutaneous absorption has provided a rational basis for the development of transdermal therapeutic systems, the objective of which has been to use the skin as a route of entry for the controlled maintained input of drugs at predetermined rates to the systemic circulation. Results of clinical studies have indicated good agreement between percutaneous absorption *in vivo* and *in vitro*.

REFERENCES

1. Shaw, J. E., Chandrasekaran, S. K., Michaels, A. S., and Taskovich, L. (1975). Controlled transdermal delivery, *in vitro* and *in vivo*. In *Animal Models in Human Dermatology*, ed. H. Maibach, p. 138. New York, Churchill-Livingstone.
2. Michaels, A. S., Chandrasekaran, S. K., and Shaw, J. E. (1975). Drug permeation through human skin: Theory and *in vitro* experimental measurement. *Am. Inst. Chem. Eng.* 21:985.
3. Chandrasekaran, S. K., Michaels, A. S., Campbell, P., and Shaw, J. E. (1976). Scopolamine permeation through human skin *in vitro*. *Am. Inst. Chem. Eng.* 22(5):828.
4. Bayne, W. F., Tao, F. T., and Crisologo, N. (1975). Submicrogram assay for scopolamine in plasma and urine. *J. Pharm. Sci.* 64:288.
5. Shaw, J. E., and Schmitt, L. G. (1976). Clinical pharmacology of scopolamine in prevention of motion-induced nausea. (In preparation.)
6. Bartek, M. J., LaBudde, J. A., and Maibach, H. I. (1972). Skin permeability *in vivo*: Comparison in rat, rabbit, pig and man. *J. Invest. Dermatol.* 48:114.

Metabolism of Cutaneously Applied Surfactants

Robert B. Drotman

Miami Valley Laboratories
The Procter and Gamble Company
Cincinnati, Ohio

The traditional way of studying the metabolism of xeno-biotics is to prepare the compound with radioactive labeling in the molecule, give a dose of the labeled compound orally to an experimental animal, measure the rate and extent of absorption, the route and rate of excretion, the amount of radioactivity retained in the carcass and selected organs, and finally to isolate and identify the biotransformation products. Sometimes parenteral administration is used, rather than oral, to eliminate questions of absorption or microbial biotransformation.

The information obtained in such studies forms the basis for extrapolating toxicological data from experimental animals to humans. It can also alert the investigator to possible accumulation of the substance in the organism, and may detect biotransformation products that warrant toxicological studies of their own apart from those of the originally-dosed substance.

Useful as such studies are, they are not altogether adequate for materials whose principal site of exposure is the skin. When a material is put on the skin it may or may not be absorbed to the same extent as when it is ingested. If left on the skin, it may continue to be absorbed for many hours or days. Moreover the material may be metabolized by skin microflora which may result in unique metabolic products for that compound.

In evaluating the toxicity of surfactants, oral toxicity *is* studied because even such products as laundry detergents are sometimes swallowed. But attention is also given to cutaneous toxicity for those surfactants that are expected to come into contact with the skin for extended times during normal use. Therefore, it is appropriate, when the expected skin contact time warrants it, to find out how surfactants are metabolized by the skin.

The methods used to study the metabolism of surfactants in our laboratories are conventional. A surfactant is synthesized with a radioisotope label in one or more positions, depending on the chemical nature of the material. The labeled material is applied to the skin of experimental animals. Urine, feces, and carbon dioxide are collected at intervals for a predetermined period of time and finally the excess substance is washed from the application site and the experimental animals sacrificed. The excreta, skin washings, various organs, and especially the skin at the application site are then assayed for radioactivity. When it is appropriate, biotransformation products are isolated and identified. Because this can be a long and expensive process, each metabolic program must be tailored individually for each substance that is to be investigated.

In some cases the metabolic studies are extended to humans. When humans volunteer for such studies appropriate safeguards are taken. The subject is dosed on a predesignated area of skin and then urine, feces, and CO_2 are collected for a predetermined period of time. At the end of the experiment alcohol- or water-saturated swabs are used to remove the remaining surfactant from the skin. In the case of human studies material balance is calculated by adding the radioactivity recovered from the excreta to that recovered from the skin.

This presentation will be limited to the specific metabolic programs for four different surfactants, of three different types: cationic, anionic, and nonionic. These programs have ranged from simple to complex.

CATIONIC SURFACTANTS

Figure 1 shows the structure of a quaternary ammonium chloride, dialkyl (octadecyl) dimethyl ammonium chloride (DADMAC), that is widely used in laundry softener products. This material will serve as an example of a cationic surfactant. For our studies, the first carbon of one alkyl group was radiolabeled with ^{14}C. Ten milligrams (~ 30 μCi) of [^{14}C]-DADMAC was applied to the back of each of four rabbits

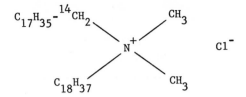

Dioctadecyl dimethyl [1-^{14}C] ammonium chloride

Fig. 1. Structure of a quaternary ammonium chloride; a cationic surfactant.

over a 5 x 8 cm area. The rabbits were then restrained for 72 hr so they could not lick the material from their backs or rub against their cages. Their excreta were collected over a 72 hr period and were assayed for radioactivity. Table 1 shows the distribution of radioactivity between excreta, test skin site, other skin, and the cage wash. Only traces of radioactivity were found in the carbon dioxide, urine, and feces; most of the radioactivity was recovered from the skin site where it had been applied. The figure of $\sim 90 \pm 10\%$ for total recovery of radioactivity is fairly typical for our experiments.

We interpreted this experiment as clear evidence that dialkyl (octadecyl) dimethyl ammonium chloride does not effectively penetrate the skin. Confirmation of this conclusion was obtained from *in vitro* experiments using human infant abdominal skin. The dialkyl (octadecyl) dimethyl ammonium chloride did not pass through this skin.

ANIONIC SURFACTANTS

Figure 2 shows the structure of an anionic surfactant that is widely used in laundry detergents, linear alkylbenzenesulfonate (LAS); this material was radiolabeled with ^{35}S. Radioactive LAS was applied to the skin of several species--rat, rabbit, guinea pig, and human--and was left in place for 72 hr (144 hr for the human). All animals were harnessed or restrained so as to prevent oral ingestion. The fate of the radioactivity was then determined. The results are presented in Table 2. Only traces of the radioactivity appeared in the urine or feces. In these experiments > 79% of the applied dose was recovered from the skin area to which it had been applied, except in the case of the human. The difference between animals and humans is believed to occur because the test site skin was removed from the animals and

TABLE 1

*Distribution of ^{14}C after Dioctadecyl Dimethyl [$1-^{14}C$]
Ammonium Chloride Was Applied to the Skin of Rabbits[a]*

Sample	% of Applied Radioactivity[b]
CO_2	0.27 ± 0.0
Urine	0.15 ± 0.0
Feces	0.16 ± 0.0
Test site skin	88 ± 2.3
Other skin	0.2 ± 0.1
Cage wash	0.29 ± 0.0
Total recovered	89 ± 2.4

[a]In all tables SEM = standard error of the mean.
[b]Mean ± SEM of four animals.

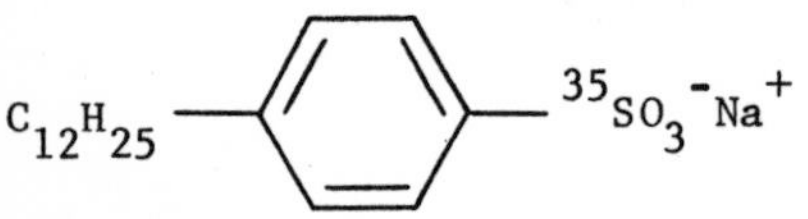

Fig. 2. Linear alkylbenzene-sulfonate (LAS); an anionic surfactant.

subjected to chemical digestion. This results in a more complete recovery of radioactive sulfur. For humans, the skin was merely swabbed, and this technique evidently did not recover material that was adsorbed to the skin. This probably accounts for the low recovery in the human study.

For both the dialkyl (octadecyl) dimethyl ammonium chloride and the LAS, the studies of cutaneous metabolism ended when it was found that the materials did not effectively penetrate the skin.

TABLE 2

Distribution of Radioactivity Found ca 72 hr after a Single Cutaneous Dose of [^{35}S]-LAS to Rats, Rabbits, Guinea Pigs, and after 144 hr in Man

	% of dose radioactivity[a]			
	Rat (n=3)	Rabbit (n=3)	Guinea Pig (n=4)	Man (n=2)[b]
Urine	0.08 ± 0.02	0.85 ± 0.02	0.20 ± 0.06	0.3, < 0.01
Feces	0.04 ± 0.02	0.38 ± 0.08	0.25 ± 0.13	0.3, 0.2
Skin app. site	92.87 ± 1.13	82.0 ± 3.6	77.80 ± 0.54	50.0, 40.8[c]
Cage wash	0.22 ± 0.08	2.02 ± 0.69	0.12 ± 0.04	
Total recovered	93.2 ± 0.88	85.3 ± 2.33	78.4 ± 0.63	51, 41

[a] Mean ± SEM for the indicated number of animals.

[b] Individual values of two subjects.

[c] This represents an application site wash only, whereas in the animal studies the radioactivity remaining at the application site was determined by complete digestion and analysis of the entire skin sample.

NONIONIC SURFACTANTS

DODECYL DIMETHYL AMINE OXIDE

The next surfactant to be considered did penetrate the skin, and a more extensive study was necessary. This surfactant was *dodecyl dimethyl amine oxide* (DDAO), an example of a nonionic surfactant, whose structure is shown in Figure 3. DDAO is used in commercial products in combination with an anionic surfactant and this may alter both the penetration and the metabolism of DDAO.

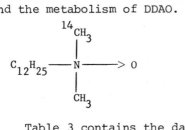

Fig. 3. *Dodecyl dimethyl amine oxide (DDAO); a nonionic surfactant.*

Table 3 contains the data from a disposition experiment in rats with [^{14}C-methyl] DDAO. Ten mg of DDAO containing 13 µCi of ^{14}C were applied as an aqueous solution to an 18 cm^2 site on the backs of 200 g rats. The rats were restrained for the duration of the experiment. The data indicate that ∿ 40% of the applied radioactivity was absorbed through the skin. The majority of the excreted radioactivity was detected in urine with lesser amounts in carbon dioxide and feces.

A relatively large fraction remained in the carcass. The radioactivity found in the carcass is at least partly a result of the dosing procedure. Table 4 shows that the appearance of radioactivity in excreta was approximately uniform throughout the 72 hr duration of the experiment. This indicates that radioactivity was being absorbed steadily from the reservoir of material lying on the skin.

The fate of topically applied DDAO was also investigated in other animal species. The pattern of distribution of DDAO was similar in the rat and the mouse, with the rabbit showing some quantitative differences in the disposition of radioactivity, as shown in Table 5. In all three species, most of the radioactivity that was absorbed was found in the urine. However, the quantitative difference in the disposition of radioactivity between the rabbit and the other two species may be related either to the manner of dosing or to species metabolic differences. The rabbit was given the same quantity of labeled DDAO as the rat, 10 mg, but it was spread over an area more than twice as large (18 versus 40 cm^2). Therefore, the opportunity for absorption was considerably greater, as might be expected. In addition, as several speakers at this conference have mentioned, rabbit skin is more highly absorptive than the skin of other species.

TABLE 3

Distribution of Radioactivity 72 hr after $[^{14}C]DDAO$ Was Applied to the Skin of Rats

Sample	% of applied radioactivity[a]
CO_2	2.5 ± 0.3
Urine	14.2 ± 1.9
Feces	1.8 + 0.2
Total excreta	18.5 ± 2.4
Liver	0.4 ± 0.1
Kidneys	0.05 ± 0.0
Carcass	15.6 + 2.7
Total tissues	16.1 ± 2.7
Test site skin	48.0 ± 3.2
Cage wash	6.1 + 1.3
Total recovered	88.8 ± 1.6

[a]Mean ± SEM; $n = 4$.

The disposition of radioactivity after dermal application of DDAO was compared with the distribution after oral dosing. More of the oral dose was absorbed than the cutaneous dose, but of the material that was absorbed, most was excreted in the urine, with smaller amounts in the carbon dioxide and feces (Table 6).

The mouse and the rabbit likewise showed similar patterns of distribution after either oral or cutaneous doses.

In order to get a better understanding of what was happening to the DDAO after it had been absorbed into the animal's body, the chemical state of the ^{14}C that was excreted in the urine was examined. For this purpose the radioactive components in urine were fractionated by cation-exchange chromatography. The fractions were counted for radioactivity and a plot of the radioactivity of material eluting from

TABLE 4

Appearance of ^{14}C in Excreta with Time After Application of $[^{14}C]DDAO$ to the Skin of Rats

Sample	% of applied radioactivity[a]		
	0-24 hr	24-48 hr	48-72 hr
CO_2	0.64 ± 0.02	0.76 ± 0.10	0.89 ± 0.17
Urine	4.5 ± 0.30	4.7 ± 1.00	5.1 ± 1.00
Feces	0.5 ± 0.08	0.8 ± 0.01	0.4 ± 0.12

[a]Mean ± SEM; n = 4.

TABLE 5

Distribution of Radioactivity 74 hr After Applying $[^{14}C]DDAO$ to the Skin of Several Species[a]

Sample	% of applied radioactivity		
	Rat[b]	Mouse[c]	Rabbit[d]
CO_2	2.5 ± 0.3	5 ± 1.0	1.4 ± 0.7
Urine	14.2 ± 1.9	11.6 ± 6.0	42.1 ± 6.3
Feces	1.8 ± 0.2	1.4 ± 0.3	2.2 ± 0.7
Tissues	15.6 ± 2.7	17.6 ± 1.7	5.1 ± 0.5
Test-site skin	48.0 ± 3.2	48.9 ± 9.5	39.4 ± 8.2
Cage wash	6.1 ± 1.3	10.6 ± 3.5	3.9 ± 2.2
Total recovered	88.8 ± 1.6	95.2 ± 5.2	94.4 ± 3.2

[a]Mean ± S.D.   [c]n = 3.
[b]n = 4.   [d]n = 4.

TABLE 6

Distribution of Radioactivity after Oral and Cutaneous Dosing of [^{14}C]DDAO to Rats

| Sample | % of administered radioactivity[a] | |
	Cutaneous dosing	Oral dosing
CO_2	2.5 ± 0.3	18 ± 1.8
Urine	14.2 ± 1.9	37.8 ± 7.1[b]
Feces	1.8 ± 0.2	21.2 ± 8.7
Bile	--	3.6 + 0.4
Total excreted	18.5 ± 2.4	80.8 ± 9.0
Carcass	15.6 ± 2.7	14.8 ± 5.8
Test-site skin	48.0 ± 3.2	--
Cage wash	6.1 + 1.3	--
Total recovered	88.8 ± 1.6	95.6 ± 5.4

[a] Mean ± SEM; $n = 4$.

[b] Includes cage wash.

the chromatograph (metabolite profile) is shown in Figure 4. The metabolite profile in Figure 4, then, describes the metabolites in urine from rats that were dosed cutaneously with DDAO labeled at the methyl position.

From such a chromatogram as this it is not possible to identify, chemically, the several peaks, and it is possible that at least some of them represent more than one substance. Nevertheless, the metabolite profile is an important tool for investigating the metabolism of compounds. For instance, we have compared this profile with the metabolite profile of rats that have been dosed orally with DDAO. The metabolite profile from urine of the orally dosed rats is qualitatively the same as that from the cutaneously dosed animals. Although there are some differences in the relative heights of the peaks, both samples showed peaks at the same retention times, indicating that the chemical changes DDAO undergoes

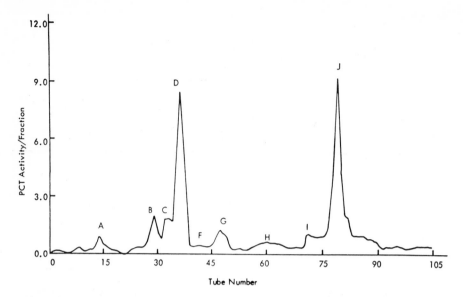

Fig. 4. *Chromatographic profile of urine from a rat dosed cutaneously with [^{14}C-methyl]DDAO.*

as it "passes through" the animal are comparable, whether the material enters through the skin or through the gut. This finding also may indicate that neither intestinal microflora nor skin microflora play a predominant role in the biotransformation of DDAO.

Another comparison of metabolite profiles has been between species. The metabolite profile for the rabbit is similar to that for the rat (Figure 4), except that in the rabbit metabolite profile, one of the peaks, labeled D, is much larger, and peak J is much smaller. From this it appears that the rat and the rabbit metabolize DDAO in similar ways, but with different ratios among the metabolites generated.

All of the work described so far was done with DDAO radiolabeled in one of the methyl groups. DDAO was also prepared with ^{14}C at the α-carbon of the alkyl chain. This material was dosed to animals and urine subsequently collected. Chromatography of the urine gave a metabolite profile similar to that obtained with the methyl-labeled DDAO. This indicates that the metabolites in this chromatogram are not a result of metabolites derived by splitting the methyl group from the molecule.

The observation that cutaneous and oral dosing gave similar profiles was fortunate, since it permitted the use of oral dosing for preparing large samples from which the metabolites could be isolated and identified. It is simpler to get large quantities of radioactive urine from orally dosed animals than from cutaneously dosed animals.

One piece of valuable information obtained from these studies is that since the metabolic patterns by cutaneous and oral routes are very similar, oral long-term dosing toxicity data also apply to the cutaneous exposure of these materials.

ALKYL POLYETHOXYLATES

The final example of surfactant metabolism I want to discuss is that of the alkyl polyethoxylates. Their general structure is $C_nH_{2n+1}(OCH_2CH_2)_mOH$, where $n = 11-15$ and $m = 4-6$ in commercial preparations. They are composed of a long hydrocarbon chain attached to a polyethoxylate unit that terminates in a hydroxyl group. These nonionic surfactants are widely used in liquid detergents. A wide range of homologous compounds is available, differing from each other in the length of the alkyl group or in the number of ethoxylate units. Most commercial products contain a mixture of homologs. We have studied the cutaneous metabolism of several of these homologs.

For our studies we have varied both the alkyl chain length and the number of ethoxylate units. In order to study these compounds thoroughly we have varied the position of the isotope label in the molecule. In the first three structures shown in Figure 5, ^{14}C was in the first carbon of the alkyl group. In the second three it was in the first carbon of the polyoxyethylene chain. For example, we designate one of these compounds as $*C_{12}E_6$, meaning a 12-carbon alkyl chain attached to a series of six ethoxylate units. The asterisk shows that ^{14}C was in the hydrocarbon chain. When the asterisk is on the E in the abbreviation, this indicates that the radiolabel

$$C_{11}H_{23}*CH_2(OCH_2CH_2)_6OH = *C_{12}E_6$$

$$C_{12}H_{25}*CH_2(OCH_2CH_2)_6OH = *C_{13}E_6$$

$$C_{14}H_{29}*CH_2(OCH_2CH_2)_7OH = *C_{15}E_7$$

$$C_{12}H_{25}(OCH_2CH_2)_5OCH_2*CH_2OH = C_{12}*E_6$$

$$C_{13}H_{27}(OCH_2CH_2)_5OCH_2*CH_2OH = C_{13}*E_6$$

$$C_{14}H_{29}(OCH_2CH_2)_6OCH_2*CH_2OH = C_{14}*E_7$$

Fig. 5. Formulas of radiolabeled alkyl polyethoxylates.

is in the ethoxylate portion of the molecule. Each of these six compounds was applied to the skin of rats and remained there for 72 hr while excreta were collected. The rats were then sacrificed, and the area of the skin where the compound had been applied was assayed for radioactivity, along with other organs of the body and the residual carcass.

Table 7 contains the disposition results of cutaneous dosing. Each of the compounds penetrated the skin. This is shown by the fact that > 20% of the ^{14}C appeared in the excretory products (urine, CO_2, feces) and the carcass. As with previous animal experiments, the rats were restrained throughout the course of the experiment to prevent oral ingestion.

When rats were dosed with the series of alkyl ethoxylates which had ^{14}C in the alkyl chain the principal route of excretion was the urine for $*C_{12}E_6$ and $*C_{13}E_6$. However, when animals were dosed cutaneously with $*C_{15}E_7$ the principal route of excretion of ^{14}C was expired CO_2. In addition, there was a statistically significant increase in the $^{14}CO_2$ from $*C_{13}E_6$ when compared to $*C_{12}E_6$. These results indicate that the amount of radioactivity appearing in CO_2 from alkyl radiolabeled alkyl ethoxylates is a function of alkyl chain length. We have, at the present time, no explanation for this metabolic difference with these homologs.

Experiments in which the radiolabel was in the ethoxylate portion of the molecule resulted in the same basic pattern of disposition for the three alkyl ethoxylates tested. The largest portion of excreted radioactivity was in the urine, with lesser amounts in CO_2 and feces.

When these six compounds were administered orally, the same basic disposition pattern as was noted with cutaneous administration was evident as seen in Table 8. Again the trend in the alkyl ethoxylates with the radiolabel in the alkyl portion of the molecule is towards greater amounts of $^{14}CO_2$ excreted with longer alkyl-chain lengths. In addition, because of the greater absorption with the orally dosed animals, less radioactivity appears in feces. The rats dosed with the radiolabel in the ethoxylate portion of the molecule all have the same basic disposition pattern. The largest portion of the excreted radioactivity is in the urine, with lesser amounts in feces and the lowest amounts in CO_2. Recovery in all these experiments was considered to be good and ranged from 87 to 90%.

The series of experiments with the alkyl ethoxylates demonstrates the value of both investigating homologs within a series and labeling the molecule at different positions to be sure that the results represent the metabolic fate of all parts of the molecule.

TABLE 7

Distribution of Radioactivity 72 hr After Cutaneous Application of Radioactive Alkyl Ethoxylate to Rats

Sample	% of administered radioactivity[a]					
	$^{*}C_{12}E_6$	$^{*}C_{13}E_6$	$^{*}C_{15}E_7$	$C_{12}{^{*}}E_6$	$C_{13}{^{*}}E_6$	$C_{14}{^{+}}E_7$
CO_2	4.2 ± 0.4	9.1 ± 1.2	21.7 ± 3.4	3.4 ± 0.2	2.3 ± 0.2	2.4 ± 0.0
Urine	23.4 ± 4.6	21.1 ± 4.3	6.4 ± 1.5	24.8 ± 8.2	15.1 ± 2.8	16.1 ± 2.0
Feces	6.2 ± 0.5	6.4 ± 0.9	1.8 ± 0.6	3.4 ± 2.3	4.9 ± 0.7	5.4 ± 0.5
Total carcass	10.2 ± 0.6	9.3 ± 1.0	11.7 ± 0.8	7.2 ± 1.3	16.6 ± 0.7	14.2 ± 1.2
Test-site skin	41.7 ± 3.2	42.4 ± 4.6	47.1 ± 8.9	59.7 ± 13.1	43.6 ± 14.1	56.9 ± 5.7
Cage wash	3.9 ± 0.7	3.1 ± 0.0	6.2 ± 4.0	2.5 ± 1.3	17.5 ± 12.6	6.6 ± 2.8
Total recovered	89.6 ± 2.2	91.4 ± 1.7	94.9 ± 1.7	101.0 ± 5.0	100 ± 5.8	101.6 ± 2.6

[a]Mean ± SEM; *n* = 4.

TABLE 8

Distribution of Radioactivity 72 hr After Oral Dosing of Radioactive Alkyl Ethoxylate to Rats

Sample	% of administered radioactivity[a]					
	$*C_{12}E_6$	$*C_{13}E_6$	$*C_{15}E_7$	$C_{12}*E_6$	$C_{13}*E_6$	$C_{14}*E_7$
CO_2	3.6 + 0.4	20.4 + 1.8	53.7 + 5.4	3.2 + 0.3	2.4 + 0.2	1.9 + 0.1
Urine	48.7 + 6.4	45.1 + 1.2	12.3 + 3.4	52.1 + 8.1	53.9 + 5.9	54.9 + 8.4
Feces	25.4 + 5.1	13.3 + 3.0	7.9 + 1.0	27.0 + 4.8	25.6 + 2.6	22.7 + 2.1
Total carcass	9.2 + 0.7	4.7 + 0.5	8.9 + 2.0	1.7 + 0.2	1.9 + 0.5	2.7 + 1.1
G.I. wash	0.8 + 0.2	1.1 + 0.5	0.2 + 0.1	0.8 + 0.2	0.6 + 0.3	0.4 + 0.2
Cage wash	2.6 + 1.0	2.2 + 0.7	3.0 + 0.9	2.4 + 1.4	1.9 + 0.5	2.9 + 1.1
Total recovered	90.3 + 2.2	86.8 + 4.8	86 + 8.2	87.2 + 3.8	86.3 + 2.5	85.5 + 7.4

[a]Mean + SEM; $n = 4$.

SUMMARY

The tools and techniques are available for studying the metabolism of surfactants that are applied epicutaneously. The results of such studies are pertinent to the toxicological evaluation of surfactants since they aid in ascertaining the degree of certainty with which one can extrapolate toxicological test data from animal to man. In the studies described here, the metabolism of surfactants that are absorbed through the skin seems generally to parallel their metabolism by the oral route.

ACKNOWLEDGMENTS

Dr. N. R. Artman aided in the preparation of this paper, and Drs. D. P. Rice, J. A. Budny, R. W. Geisler, F. A. Hartman, and T. S. Turan provided some of the information presented.

Percutaneous Absorption in Man and Animal:
A Perspective

Ronald C. Wester

Research Division, Searle Laboratories,
Chicago, Illinois,

Howard I. Maibach

Department of Dermatology
University of California School of Medicine,
San Francisco, California

Our objective is to compare percutaneous absorption in various animal models with the absorption that occurs in human skin. Our discussion will be limited to studies involving actual comparisons between animal and human skin, and data relative to *in vivo* and *in vitro* models per se will not be reviewed.

COMPARISON OF *IN VIVO* STUDIES

The basic data for *in vivo* human percutaneous absorption, to which animal models will be compared, were obtained from publications of Feldmann and Maibach (1, 2, 3). In these clinical studies a specific concentration of radioactive compound (4 $\mu g/cm^2$) was applied to a specific anatomical site (ventral forearm); the area was not occluded and subjects were requested not to wash the area for 24 hr. Urine was collected for 5 days, divided into suitable time periods, and assayed for radioactivity. A tracer dose was also given parenterally, and the percent radioactivity in the urine following parenteral administration was then used to correct for compound which might be excreted by some other route and for compound which might be retained within the body. Data from these clinical studies will be compared with the results obtained in other studies.

Bartek *et al.* (4) undertook a comparative study of percutaneous absorption in rats, rabbits, miniature swine, and
man. Methodology in the animals was similar to that in man,
except that in animals the compounds were applied to the skin
of the back. Table 1 compares the results obtained with
pertinent data from Feldmann and Maibach (1, 2). Haloprogin,
a topical antifungal agent, was completely absorbed in the
rat and rabbit. Penetration through the skin of pigs and
man was similar and much slower than it was through rat and
rabbit skin. Penetration of acetylcysteine was minimal in
all species. Cortisone, a minimal penetrant through the skin
of man and miniature swine, was well absorbed in the rat and
rabbit. Caffeine readily penetrated the skin of all species.
With butter yellow, penetration through rabbit skin was much
greater than through the skin of the other three species.
Testosterone penetration, which will be discussed later, was
also studied. The results of this study, summarized in
Figure 1, show rabbit skin to be the most permeable to topically applied compounds, followed closely by rat skin. In
contrast, it appears that the permeability of the skin of
the miniature swine is closer to that of human skin.

A comparison of percutaneous absorption in the rhesus
monkey and in man was made by Wester and Maibach (5, 6).
Methodology and the site of application (ventral forearm)
were the same for both species. Hydrocortisone, testosterone, and benzoic acid in the monkey showed the same low,
middle, and high absorption, respectively, as in man. Since
Bartek *et al.* (4) used the same design to compare penetration in the rat, rabbit, and pig, their data on testosterone
penetration can also be used for comparison with the monkey.
Combining the data shows that of all the species studied,
absorption of testosterone in the rhesus monkey was closest
to that in the human (Figure 2).

Bartek and La Budde (7) studied the percutaneous absorption of pesticides in the rabbit, pig, and squirrel monkey
and compared the results with the absorption obtained in
man (3). As demonstrated in Table 2, DDT was a minimal
penetrant in man, whereas in the rabbit and pig penetration
rates were considerably greater. Absorption in the squirrel
monkey was very low; however, the value reported was uncor-
rected with parenteral control data. Penetration of lindane,
parathion, and malathion in the rabbit exceeded that in the
other species. With lindane, penetration in the squirrel
monkey was closer to that in man, whereas with parathion
penetration in the pig was closest to that in man. Penetration of malathion was similar in the squirrel monkey and the
pig, and could be predictive of that in man. It may be concluded that the *in vivo* percutaneous absorption of pesticides in the rabbit was much greater than in man, whereas

TABLE 1

Percutaneous Absorption of Several Compounds by Rat, Rabbit, Pig, and Man (in Vivo) [a]

| Penetrant | Percent of dose absorbed (+SD) [b] | | | |
	Rat	Rabbit	Pig	Man
Haloprogin	95.8 + 13.9	113.0 + 16.5	19.7 + 9.9	11.0 + 3.7
Acetylcysteine	3.5 + 3.8	2.0 + 1.0	6.0	2.4 + 1.6
Cortisone	24.7 + 3.6	30.3 + 9.0	4.1 + 1.6	3.4 + 1.6
Caffeine	53.1 + 11.8	69.2 + 5.8	32.4 + 4.8	47.6 + 20.9
Butter yellow	48.2 + 2.2	100.0 + 7.9	41.9 + 10.0	21.6 + 4.9
Testosterone	47.4 + 2.6	69.6 + 7.8	29.4 + 8.6	13.2 + 3.0

[a] Data from Bartek et al. (4) and Feldmann and Maibach (1, 2).

[b] Corrected for recovery following parenteral administration.

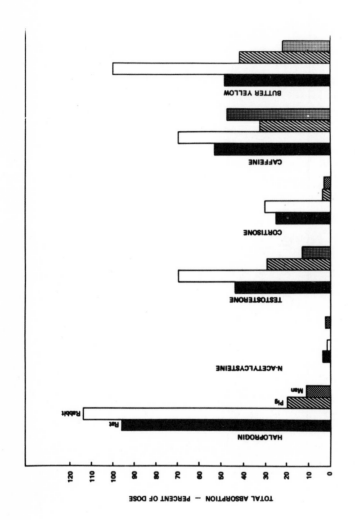

Fig. 1. Percutaneous absorption of several compounds by rat, rabbit, miniature swine, and man. Rabbit skin in vivo was most permeable to topically applied compounds, followed closely by rat skin. The permeability of miniature swine skin was closer to that of human skin. (Reproduced from Bartek et al. (4), with permission of the Williams & Wilkins Co.)

114

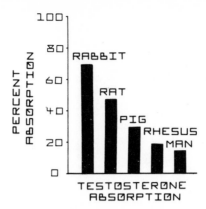

Fig. 2. Percutaneous absorption of testosterone (4 μg/cm^2) by rabbit, rat, miniature swine, rhesus monkey, and man. Penetration in the rhesus monkey was closest to that in man. [Data from Bartek et al. (4) and Wester and Maibach (5).]

penetration in the pig and squirrel monkey was closer to that in man.

Further evidence of the similarity of skin penetration in the rhesus monkey and man was shown by Wester and Maibach (8) in their studies of the relationship of topical dose and percutaneous absorption. As shown in Table 3, the *in vivo* percutaneous absorption of testosterone, hydrocortisone, and benzoic acid was similar for the rhesus monkey and man. Also, the dose-response was similar in the two species. There are two important points in this study. First, the efficiency of absorption (percent) as well as the mass of material absorbed (μg) changed as the topical dose changed, as illustrated in Figure 3. This relationship will be noted again when the results from *in vitro* studies are compared. Secondly, and more important to our present discussion, this relationship of topical dose to absorption is similar in the rhesus monkey and man for the three compounds studied (Figure 4).

Hunziker *et al.* (9) studied the percutaneous absorption of ^{14}C-labeled benzoic acid, progesterone, and testosterone in the Mexican hairless dog, and compared the absorption with that obtained in man. Total absorption and maximum absorption rates were greater in man than in the hairless dog. Surface counting experiments showed that benzoic acid and progesterone persisted on the dog skin far longer than on human skin.

In general, the comparative *in vivo* data which have been reviewed demonstrate that percutaneous absorption in the pig

TABLE 2

Percutaneous Absorption of Several Pesticides by Rabbit, Pig, Squirrel Monkey, and Man (in Vivo)[a]

Pesticide	Percent of dose absorbed (+SD)[b]			
	Rabbit	Pig	Monkey	Man
DDT	46.3 + 1.4	43.4 + 7.9	1.5 + 2.0[c]	10.4 + 3.6
Lindane	51.2 + 29.9	37.6 + 2.8	16.0 + 10.9	9.3 + 3.7
Parathion	97.5 + 8.0	14.5 + 0.8	30.3 + 10.5	9.7 + 5.9
Malathion	64.6 + 11.4	15.5 + 2.5	19.3 + 2.1	8.2 + 2.7

[a]Data from Bartek and La Budde (7) and Feldmann and Maibach (3).

[b]Corrected for recovery following parenteral administration.

[c]Not corrected with parenteral dose.

TABLE 3

*Percutaneous Absorption of Increased Topical Doses of
Several Compounds in the Rhesus Monkey and Man (in Vivo)[a]*

| Penetrant | Dose, $\mu g/cm^2$ | Percent of dose absorbed ($\pm$SD)[b] | |
		Rhesus	Man
Hydrocortisone	4	2.9 + 0.8	1.9 + 1.6
	40	2.1 + 0.6	0.6 + 0.3
Benzoic Acid[c]	4	59.2 + 7.6	42.6 + 16.4
	40	33.6 + 5.1	25.7 + 9.9
	2000	17.4 + 1.2	14.4 + 3.8
Testosterone	4	18.4 + 9.5	13.2 + 3.0
	40	6.7 + 4.2	8.8 + 2.0[d]
	250	2.9 + 1.4	--
	400	2.2 + 1.0	2.8 + 0.9
	1600	2.9 + 1.7	--
	4000	1.4 + 0.8	--

[a]Data from Wester and Maibach (5, 6, 8).

[b]Corrected for recovery following parenteral administration.

[c]Not corrected with parenteral dose.

[d]$30 \ \mu g/cm^2$.

and monkey (rhesus and squirrel) is in most cases similar to
that in man, whereas in the rat, and especially in the rabbit, skin penetration is greater than that observed in man.
The skin of the Mexican hairless dog has significantly different permeability characteristics than human skin.

COMPARISON OF HUMAN *IN VITRO* AND *IN VIVO* STUDIES

Excised skin diffusion cells may be used to study *in
vitro* percutaneous absorption. The validity of this procedure depends on three assumptions (10): (i) that no
living process affects the skin's impermeability, (ii) that
the dermis does not affect penetration, and (iii) that the
skin surface conditions of the excised system are similar to
those in life. Tregear (10) further states that because one

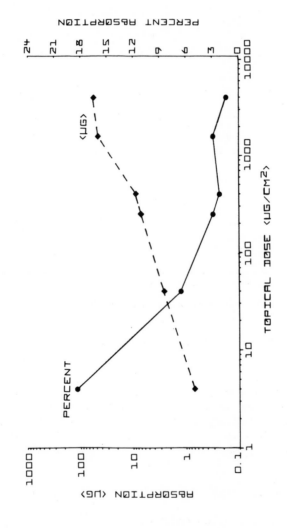

Fig. 3. Percutaneous absorption of increasing topical doses of testosterone in the rhesus monkey. The efficiency (percent) of absorption as well as the mass (μg) of material absorbed changed as the topical dose changed. [Reproduced from Wester and Maibach (8), with permission of the Williams & Wilkins Co.]

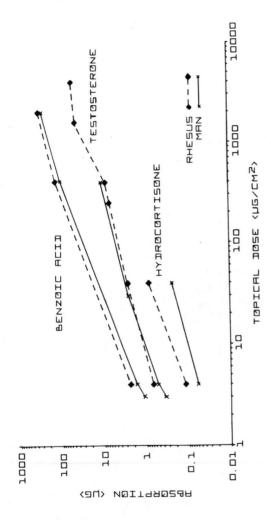

Fig. 4. Comparison between rhesus monkey and man of compounds absorbed (µg) after topical application of increasing doses (µg/cm²) of
testosterone, hydrocortisone, and benzoic acid. The topical dose
response of the three compounds was similar for the rhesus monkey and
man. [Reproduced from Wester and Maibach (8), with permission of the
Williams & Wilkins Co.]

can rarely, if ever, be certain that these assumptions are completely justified, it is always desirable to check important findings *in vivo*.

Most pertinent to this discussion is the work of Franz (11) on the relevance of *in vitro* data. He evaluated the permeability of 12 organic compounds *in vitro* using excised human skin and compared the results to those obtained previously by Feldmann and Maibach in living man (2). Care was taken to insure that his *in vitro* conditions closely followed those used *in vivo*, although it was necessary to use human abdominal skin for the *in vitro* studies. Additionally, the doses employed ranged from 4 to 40 $\mu g/cm^2$, with the assumption that the percent of applied dose absorbed would not be dose dependent.

The results obtained in the *in vivo* and *in vitro* studies are shown in Table 4. Quantitatively, the two sets of data do not agree. The *in vitro* method was of value to the extent that it tended to distinguish compounds of low permeability from those of high permeability. However, there are notable differences such that the *in vitro* method alone would not always be a reliable or accurate predictor of percutaneous absorption in living man. The *in vitro* method did accurately show the kinetics of absorption as seen *in vivo* for the 12 compounds. Factors which make such quantitative analysis by the *in vitro* method so difficult are the difference in absorption depending on the site of application (12) and the absence of desquamation in excised skin. Additionally, the assumption that the percent of applied dose absorbed would be the same over the dose range of 4 to 40 $\mu g/cm^2$ clearly is not warranted for all compounds, as shown in Table 3 and Figures 3 and 4.

COMPARISON OF *IN VITRO* STUDIES

Table 5 summarizes the ranking of skin permeability of different species, as determined *in vitro* by various investigators (10, 13, 14). Allowing for the different compounds used in each study to rank the species and the differences in origin of the skin sample (back, forearm), the studies generally show that the skin of common laboratory animals (rabbit, rat, and guinea pig) is more permeable than the skin of man. Skin from the pig and the monkey more generally approximates the permeability of human skin. Not surprisingly, this general ranking is in close agreement with the *in vivo* data discussed earlier.

Campbell *et al.* (15) recently investigated the permeation of scopolamine *in vitro* through rat, rabbit, and human skin. The results indicated that human skin is the least

TABLE 4

Percutaneous Absorption of Several Compounds by Human Skin in Vivo and in Vitro[a]

Compound	Percent of dose absorbed	
	in Vivo[b]	in Vitro[c]
Hippuric acid	0.2 ± 0.1	1.2 (0.8, 2.7)
Nicotinic acid	0.3 ± 0.1	3.3 (0.7, 8.3)
Thiourea	0.9 ± 0.2	3.4 (2.4, 5.5)
Chloramphenicol	2.0 ± 2.5	2.9 (1.0, 5.7)
Phenol	4.4 ± 2.4	10.9 (7.7, 26)
Urea	6.0 ± 1.9	11.1 (5.2, 29)
Nicotinamide	11.1 ± 6.2	28.8 (16, 65)
Acetylsalicylic acid	21.8 ± 3.1	40.5 (17, 49)
Salicylic acid	22.8 ± 13.2	12.0 (2.3, 23)
Benzoic acid	42.6 ± 16.5	44.9 (29, 53)
Caffeine	47.6 ± 21.0	9.0 (5.5, 20)
Dinitrochlorobenzene	53.1 ± 12.4	27.5 (19, 33)

[a]Data from Franz (11), with permission of the Williams & Wilkins Co.

[b]Mean value (±SD).

[c]Median value (95% confidence interval).

permeable of the three species tested, and the relative order of rat and rabbit skin permeabilities depends both on skin location (back and side) and the method used to remove the hair.

In the study of Marzulli *et al.* (13) mouse skin was the most permeable, and was certainly much more permeable than human skin. In contrast, penetration of human and hairless

TABLE 5

Ranking of Skin Permeability of Different Species as Determined in Vitro, *Listed in Decreasing Order of Permeability*

Tregear (10)	Marzulli *et al.* (13)	McGreesh (14)
rabbit	mouse	rabbit
rat	guinea pig	rat
guinea pig	goat	guinea pig
man	rabbit	cat
	horse	goat
	cat	monkey
	dog	dog
	monkey	pig
	weanling pig	
	man	
	chimpanzee	

mouse skin *in vitro* appears to be similar (16). Table 6 shows the *in vitro* penetration of several compounds through skin of the two species.

The chief advantage of diffusion cells over the use of intact animals or men is the ease of measurement of the penetrant. This then provides a model whereby different compounds can be screened or different preparations of a compound can be directly compared, as shown in Table 6 for 1% thiabendazole. However, the final conclusions should be based on *in vivo* data, preferably in man or in a species relevant to man.

GENERAL COMMENTS

This summary, complete for our present state of

TABLE 6

Percutaneous Absorption of Human and Hairless Mouse Skin (in Vitro)[a]

	Percent absorbed	
Penetrant	Human	Hairless mouse
[^{3}H] betamethasone-17-valerate 0.001 M	0.7	0.8
[^{3}H] betamethadone alcohol 0.001 M	0.7	0.9
[^{14}C] tolnaftate 0.5%	0.9	1.4
[^{14}C] hydrocortisone alcohol	1.3	1.9
[^{14}C] 5-fluorouracil	14.2	16.1
[^{14}C] Fluocinolone acetonide 0.001 M	6.4	7.7
[^{14}C] Fluocinilone acetonide acetate 0.001 M	4.4	5.5
[^{14}C] thiabendazole 0.5%	9.4	14.6
1% Thiabendazole in:		
Dimethylacetamide	9.4	14.6
Gel base	0.7	1.3
USP hydrophilic ointment	0.1	0.3

[a] Data from Stoughton (16).

knowledge, presents only the obvious comparisons. As more is learned of the relevance of pharmacokinetics to pharmacological and toxicologic effects this aspect will be profitably reexamined. Some compounds may have similar total penetration in two species, but different metabolism and pharmacokinetics.

Many technical variables must still be examined to aid

in more relevant experimental design. Although we have a general survey on the striking anatomic regional differences of percutaneous penetration in man, we have no similar geographic atlas for the commonly employed experimental animals (17). It is possible that certain anatomic sites in an animal may be relevant to the same or another site in man. It is also likely that important regional differences exist in animals as they do in man.

In animal experiments a problem of considerable importance is that of contamination by the chemical's falling off or being removed from the skin surface when metabolism cages are used. This source of error can be controlled in the monkey if the animal is placed in a metabolism chair and the arms are prevented from moving with reinforced adhesive tape. The site of application, the ventral forearm, is isolated from the urine and fecal collection area (5). A practical and convenient alternative is to employ urinary catheters. Contamination is also avoided when a special nonocclusive protective device is utilized; details of construction of a device suitable for the pig are described by Bartek *et al.* (4). Similar devices must be designed for other experimental animals.

It has been commonly assumed that shaving skin greatly damages the stratum corneum and produces an increase in percutaneous absorption. An example of this is the immediate blanching seen after application of some vasoconstrictors to the shaved but not to the unshaved human forearm. It is not known whether or not shaving will affect the results obtained in pharmacokinetic studies in animals and man. The one experiment available compares percutaneous penetration of testosterone on the shaved and unshaved forearm of the rhesus monkey (5). In this instance no significant difference in penetration was noted. Additional experiments are needed to verify this point, and these should include not only different animals but also different methods of physical depilation (clipping, safety razor, electric razor) and several methods of chemical depilation.

Percutaneous penetration is a complex affair consisting of at least ten separate but interrelated processes (18). It is quite possible that there will be similarities in some steps and dissimilarities in others when comparing animal to man. In time we must develop comparative data on all the steps; for example, the metabolism of a compound may be so different as to make the measurement of flux almost irrelevant.

In all validating animal studies it is necessary to make comparisons at each stage of the penetration process. Although it is tempting to make broad generalizations early, it is obvious that too rigid a generalization with relatively minimal comparative data may be counterproductive.

SUMMARY

Comparative studies *in vivo* on percutaneous absorption have shown the skin of monkey and pig to be most relevant to the skin of man. The skin of the rabbit and rat was highly permeable when compared to human skin, and the skin of the Mexican hairless dog had permeability characteristics different than human skin.

Comparative studies *in vitro* also show that the skin of rabbit, rat, and guinea pig was more permeable than that of human skin. Skin from the pig and monkey more generally approximates the permeability of human skin.

Quantitative *in vitro* percutaneous absorption in human skin was not in agreement with *in vivo* penetration in man. The kinetic data do, however, show qualitative agreement.

REFERENCES

1. Feldmann, R. J., and Maibach, H. I. (1969). Percutaneous penetration of steroids in man. *J. Invest. Dermatol. 52*:89.
2. Feldmann, R. J., and Maibach, H. I. (1970). Absorption of some organic compounds through the skin in man. *J. Invest. Dermatol. 54*:399.
3. Feldmann, R. J., and Maibach, H. I. (1974). Percutaneous penetration of some pesticides and herbicides in man. *Toxicol. Appl. Pharmacol. 28*:126.
4. Bartek, M. J., La Budde, J. A., and Maibach, H. I. (1972). Skin permeability *in vivo*: Comparison in rat, rabbit, pig and man. *J. Invest. Dermatol. 58*:114.
5. Wester, R. C., and Maibach, H. I. (1975). Percutaneous absorption in the rhesus monkey compared to man. *Toxicol. Appl. Pharmacol. 32*:394.
6. Wester, R. C., and Maibach, H. I. (1975). Rhesus monkey as an animal model for percutaneous absorption. In *Animal Models in Dermatology,* ed. H. Maibach, p. 133. New York, Churchill Livingstone.
7. Bartek, M. J., and La Budde, J. A. (1975). Percutaneous absorption *in vitro*. In *Animal Models in Dermatology,* ed. H. Maibach, p. 103. New York, Churchill Livingstone.
8. Wester, R. C., and Maibach, H. I. (1976). Relationship of topical dose and percutaneous absorption in rhesus monkey and man. *J. Invest. Dermatol. 67*:518.

9. Hunziker, N., Feldmann, R. J., and Maibach, H. I. (1976). Animal models of percutaneous penetration: Comparison in Mexican hairless dogs and man. *Dermatologica* (in press).

10. Tregear, R. T. (1966). *Physical Functions of Skin*. New York, Academic Press.

11. Franz, T. J. (1975). Percutaneous absorption. On the relevance of *in vitro* data. *J. Invest. Dermatol.* *64*: 190.

12. Feldmann, R. J., and Maibach, H. I. (1967). Regional variation in percutaneous penetration of ^{14}C cortisol in man. *J. Invest. Dermatol.* *48*:181.

13. Marzulli, F. N., Brown, D. W. C., and Maibach, H. I. (1969). Techniques for studying skin penetration. *Toxicol. Appl. Pharmacol. Suppl. 3*, p. 76.

14. McGreesh, A. H. (1965). Percutaneous toxicity. *Toxicol. Appl. Pharmacol. Suppl. 2*, p. 20.

15. Campbell, P., Watanabe, T., and Chandrasekaran, S. K. (1976). Comparison of *in vitro* skin permeability of scopolamine in rat, rabbit, and man. *Fed. Proc., Fed. Am. Soc. Exp. Biol. 35*:639.

16. Stoughton, R. B. (1975). Animal models for *in vitro* percutaneous absorption. In *Animal Models in Dermatology*, ed. H. Maibach, p. 121. New York, Churchill Livingstone.

17. Maibach, H. I., Feldmann, R. J., Milby, T. H., and Serat, W. F. (1971). Regional variation in percutaneous penetration in man. *Arch. Environ. Health* *23*: 208.

18, Maibach, H. I. (1976). Ten steps to percutaneous penetration. In *Advances in Toxicology,* eds. F. Marzulli and H. Maibach. Washington, D.C., Hemisphere (in press).

The Chamber-Scarification Test
for Assessing Irritancy
of Topically Applied Substances

Peter J. Frosch and Albert M. Kligman

Department of Dermatology, Duhring Laboratories
University of Pennsylvania School of Medicine
Philadelphia, Pennsylvania

Safety requirements are becoming ever more stringent. The combined activities of consumer movements and regulatory agencies have imposed on manufacturers of topical drugs, cosmetics, and toiletries a greater burden of responsibility for alerting the user to possible harm. In consequence, the volume of materials to be tested has greatly increased. The exigencies of the current situation make it necessary to have at hand procedures which can quickly and sensitively evaluate potentially irritating chemicals and products. While animal tests are useful for screening, human assay is required to assure that the findings are relevant to man's unique integument.

The methods now in vogue are no longer adequate (1, 2, 3). Many criticisms can be leveled: (i) they take too long, the more rigorous ones requiring 10 to 21 days of continuous exposure; extended tests are costly; (ii) they are tedious and troublesome for the tester and the testee; dressings must be reapplied daily; (iii) the test substance is presented to the skin via the patch test, an archaic device which in our opinion deserves a decent burial. Patches have numerous disadvantages. Uniform exposure is difficult to attain because the patches often slide or become folded through skin movements. Reproducibility and accuracy are strongly compromised since the test material cannot be completely confined; it frequently escapes to the surrounding skin, thus lessening the concentration. Patch-testing is at best semiquantitative. (iv) Perhaps the most serious limitation of current methods is lack of sensitivity. The latter judgment requires an explanation, for previous procedures have, of course, been useful.

Irritancy is purely relative. Every substance is capable of becoming toxic for some persons under some circumstances. We are concerned with comparing agents on a scale which encompasses all materials, including ones ordinarily considered innocuous. For appraising systemic toxicity convenient measurements with clear-cut end-points are at hand, such as the LD_{50}. A dose can be found that kills 50% of experimental animals tested, and all substances can be ranked on the same scale of toxicity. The difficulty with placing topical materials on the toxicologic ladder is that application to normal skin often produces no change; accordingly, the potential toxicity of very mild irritants cannot be easily assessed.

The problem is far from a theoretical one. People differ enormously in their susceptibility to potentially toxic substances. Some have hyper-irritable integuments which are damaged by exposures that produce no changes in the majority. The reactivity of skin is influenced by many factors, viz., race, age, and the presence of cutaneous abnormalities. The latter may be very subtle. For example, the facial skin of adult Caucasoids will nearly always have been damaged by sunlight. The uninvolved skin of patients with widespred chronic dermatoses is not really normal, for clinicians have long realized that such skin can be inflamed by patch tests with substances that cause no reactions in healthy persons. Moreover, some regions of the body such as the face, scrotum, and anticubital area, are far more reactive than others such as the lower legs or palms. What might be safe for one region will not be tolerated by another. A test method will be unsatisfactory unless it takes these variables into account.

We need to know a good deal more about how to identify persons with vulnerable skins. Meanwhile we must have more dependable methods for rating materials that have weak irritancy potential. This holds true especially for cosmetics and toiletries which are used for indefinitely long periods by millions and which, unlike drugs, are required to be virtually without risk. Then too, cosmetics are often used as home treatments for a variety of minor skin problems. A reaction rate of 1 in 2,000 entails too many liabilities for the manufacturer of moisturizing creams. Premarket usage testing cannot be carried out on a scale which will allow statisticians to assess the probability within the usual confidance limits that the reaction rate will not be intolerable.

The procedure we devised earlier (the 10-day, 10-subject patch-test) is inadequate to the task (1). Subsequent experience has compelled this conclusion. To give an example: certain "moisturizing" creams caused no reactions, even when the occlusive, daily exposure was extended to 21 days and the number of subjects increased to 25. Yet we encountered women who said that their face would break out after using these very creams, testimony which we at first ignored. Putting the matter to test established the credibility of these women, at the same time rudely demonstrating to us the insensitivity of the method. Other disconcerting examples turned up with antiperspirants, antifungals and cleansing creams.

We set ourselves the tasks of: (i) replacing the patch as a vehicle of exposure and (ii) shortening the test procedure. To accomplish the latter it was necessary to create conditions which would assure the rapid penetration of the test material into the living skin. We experimented at length with various ways of breaching the horny layer barrier, including Scotch[R] tape stripping, abrasion with hard particles, pretreatment with anionic surfactants, and use of vehicles (DMSO) which promote diffusion. None of these proved feasible; the greatest problem was with reproducibility. In addition, the provoked inflammatory reactions were often intense enough to obscure the response to the test agent. We finally decided upon an ancient technique, *scarification*.

METHODS

We designed various devices for making shallow, criss-cross incisions in a reproducible fashion. None of these were as satisfactory as a deft technician using a 30-gauge half-inch needle. Individual skins are so different that mechanical gadgetry produces incisions that vary too much in depth. Eight criss-cross scratches were made with just enough pressure to cleave the epidermis but just short of drawing blood. Larger needles are difficult to control and frequently cause bleeding. The needle is held between the fingers and is drawn firmly across the skin at a 45° angle with the bevel vertical to the skin surface, that is, sideways rather than up or down (Figure 1). Holding the needle this way produces fine slits. One can soon learn to judge the proper depth by verifying the presence of sharp clefts when the skin is stretched. We found that four scratches at right angles, eight in all, gave more repeatable results than a simple cross of two scratches.

The test substances were applied to the skin within an

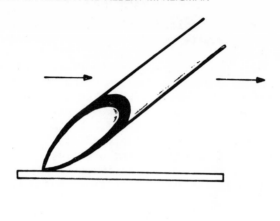

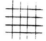

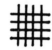

1+   Erythema confined
to scratches.

2+   Broader bands of
increased erythema with
or without rows of
vesicles, pustules or
erosions.

3+   Severe erythema
with partial confluency
with or without other
lesions.

4+   Confluent, severe
erythema sometimes
associated with edema,
necrosis or bulla
formation.

*Fig. 1.   Top, position of needle for scarifying skin.   The
bevel faces sideways and the needle is at a 45° angle.
Bottom, scoring system.*

aluminum chamber having an inner diameter of 12 mm and an
elevated flange of 2 mm (Figure 2).   Fixed quantities of the
test agents were applied, namely, 100 µg (0.1 mg) of ointments, creams, and powders, while for liquids 100 µl were
pipetted onto a disc or two thicknesses of nonwoven cotton

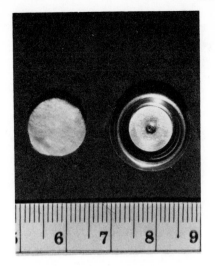

Fig. 2. The Duhring Chamber. The cloth disc is used for liquids.

cloth (Webril) snugly fitted into the chamber. The chambers were sealed to the skin by water-permeable, nonocclusive tape (Elastoplast or Dermicel). We have termed this device the Duhring Chamber. It is rather similar in design to the one created by Pirilä in Finland to replace conventional patches in tests of contact allergy (4). Pirilä's chamber (8 mm inner diameter) does not hold enough material for our purposes, having about one-tenth the capacity. Allergic reactions can be elicited by an amount of test substance far less than that required to produce irritation. Chambers have considerable advantages. The system is standardizable and markedly reduces variability. The exposure can be quantified since loss of material is prevented. The skin is in uniform contact with the test substance, which is evenly distributed. Completeness of the seal is verified at the time of removal by the presence of a circular indentation of the skin. Tape reactions are greatly lessened since occlusive tapes are not required. The diminutive size of the chamber permits exposures of up to eight substances per midvolar forearm (Figure 3). We routinely encircle the forearm with tape to assure stability. Though the back with its more permeable barrier is more reactive than the forearm (5), securement is more difficult; moreover, forearm placement is more comfortable for the subjects.

The test material was applied once daily for 3 days with daily readings. The 72 hr reading, made 30 min after removal, was the one used for calculations. The values given in the tables are mean scores. The reactions were graded on a five-point scale from 0 to 4 according to severity, as illustrated in Figures 1 and 4. With materials that evoke no

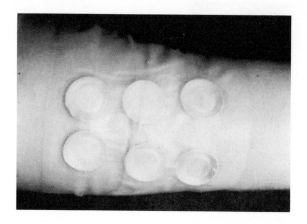

Fig. 3. Six chambers held in place with nonocclusive tape.

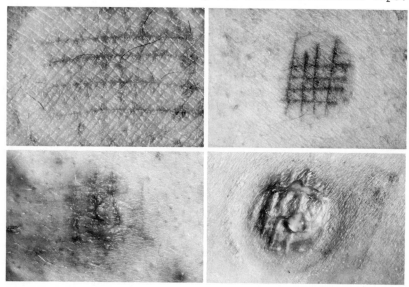

Fig. 4. Illustration of irritant reactions scored 1, 2, 3, and 4 respectively.

reaction one can barely make out the scratch marks at the end of 3 days. Five young, white college students, males and females, constituted a panel.

RESULTS

COMPARISON OF IRRITATION ON NORMAL AND SCARIFIED SKIN

For this portion of our studies we deliberately selected substances that would produce an irritant reaction within 3 days on normal skin. By determining the mean irritancy thresholds on scarified and normal skin of the same person the enhancement of sensitivity conferred by scarification can be immediately grasped. We designate the ratio of the two readings as the scarification index (SI). SIs for a score of substances are shown in Table 1.

The SI will usually exceed 10 for water-soluble chemicals that diffuse poorly through the horny layer. These substances damage normal skin only at quite high concentrations. Aluminum chloride and potassium iodide are good examples. Aluminum chloride penetrates so poorly that even under ideal *in vitro* conditions detection within the dermis is very difficult (6). However, once having entered the skin through some defect, aluminum chloride can provoke a brisk inflammatory response, as early manufacturers of antiperspirants found out. Other electrolytes such as nickel sulfate behave similarly. With nickel salts, concentrations of 20% produce marginal reactions on normal skin while 1/20 that concentration causes rows of pustules in scarified skin. Recently, Japanese workers showed that patch tests with 5% nickel sulfate provoked pustular reactions on the diseased skin of patients with atopic dermatitis, while uninvolved skin did not react at all (7). Thus, with many electrolytes conventional patch-testing may fail to disclose the potential for irritation.

The nonionic surfactants triethanolamine and Triton X-100 have very high SIs because irritation of normal skin can only be attained with concentrations of 50% and higher. Mezel's observations are pertinent with regard to the inadequacy of patch tests for detecting the irritancy potential of nonionic surfactants (8). The application of 10% Polysorbate 85 to rabbit skin for 4 days produced no visible reaction; yet an appreciable change had occurred, for the phospholipid content was increased by at least 32%. Mezei concludes that nonionic surfactants, commonly believed to be inert, may have acquired such status because of inadequate test procedures. In the scarification test, 5% Polysorbate 85 was irritating (Table 2).

Low SIs are characteristic of fairly toxic, readily penetrating lipoid-soluble irritants; hexachlorophene with an SI of 2.5 is a good example.

It should be clearly realized that SIs are not useful for grading irritants. Mild and strong irritants may have

TABLE 1

Scarification Indices

Agent	Solvent	Threshold concentration (%):		SI
		Normal skin	Scarified skin	
Surfactants				
Isostearamidopropyl morpholine lactate (1)	water	25.0	2.5	10
Stearamidopropyl dimethylamine lactate (2)	water	10.0	0.5	20
Triethanolamine	ethanol	100.0	5.0	20
Octoxynol – 9 (3)	water	50.0	1.0	50
Sodium lauryl sufate	water	0.5	0.05	10
Inorganic Salts				
Nickel sulfate	water	20.0	0.13	154
Aluminum chloride	water	30.0	2.5	12
Potassium iodide	water	60.0	5.0	12

Antimicrobials

Formalin	water	2.0	0.05	40
Triclosan (4)	ethanol	1.5	0.25	6
Benzalkonium chloride	water	0.2	0.05	4
Hexachlorophene	ethanol	2.5	1.0	2.5

Acids

Benzoic acid	ethanol	30.0	7.5	4
Lauric acid	ethanol	4.0	1.0	4
Linoleic acid	ethanol	20.0	5.0	4
Oleic acid	ethanol	30.0	5.0	6

Key to references: (1) Richamate ISML (Richardson); (2) Richamate 3780 (Richardson); (3) Triton X-100 (Rohm & Haas); (4) Irgasan DP 300 (Ciba-Geigy).

TABLE 2

Irritancy Ratings of Topical Materials

Agent	Concentration %	Vehicle	Low (0-0.4)	Slight (0.5-1.4)	Moderate (1.5-2.4)	Marked (2.5-4.0)
				Classification		
Antiperspirants						
Aluminum chloride (AlCl$_3$ 6H$_2$O)	2.5	Water		*		
	5.0	Water				* (P++)
Aluminum chlorhydroxide	50.0	Water	*			
Aluminum bromhydroxide	30.0	Water	*			
Zirconium hydroxychloride	15.0	Water			*	
Acids						
Stearic acid	25.0	Ethanol	*			
Palmitic acid	25.0	Ethanol		*		
Linoleic acid	25.0	Ethanol			*	

Compound	Conc. (%)	Solvent				
Myristic acid	25.0	Ethanol			*	
Benzoic acid	7.5	Ethanol				
	15.0	Ethanol			*	* (Er++)
Lauric acid	1.0	Ethanol				
	6.0	Ethanol			*	* (P+++)
Linoleic acid	5.0	Ethanol		*		
	12.5	Ethanol				* (Er++)
Oleic acid	5.0	Ethanol			*	
	25.0	Ethanol				
Antimicrobials						
Boric acid	5.0	Water-ethanol (1:1)	*			
Chlorhexidine	0.5	Water	*			
Hexachlorophene	1.0	Ethanol		*		
	5.0	Ethanol				* (Er++)
Triclosan (1)	0.25	Ethanol		*	*	
	1.0	Ethanol				* (Er++)
Quaternium - 1 (2)	0.1	Water			*	
	0.25	Water				* (P+++)

TABLE 2 - *continued*

Irritancy Ratings of Topical Materials

Agent	Concentration %	Vehicle	Classification			
			Low (0-0.4)	Slight (0.5-1.4)	Moderate (1.5-2.4)	Marked (2.5-4.0)
Benzalkonium chloride	0.05	Water		*		
	0.1	Water				* (P+++)
Formalin	0.05	Water		*		
	0.5	Water				* (P+++)
Urea	7.5	Water		*		
	30.0	Water				*
Basic fuchsin	1.0	Water	*			
Neomycin sulfate	2.0	Water	*			
Glutaraldehyde	2.0	Water				*
Gentian violet	1.0	Water		*		

Solvents

Solvents						
Diethylene glycol	Neat		*			
Isopropyl myristate	Neat		*			
Isopropyl palmitate	Neat			*		
Oleyl alcohol	25.0	Mineral oil	*			
Hexadecyl alcohol	25.0	Mineral oil		*		
Tetradecyl alcohol	25.0	Mineral oil			*	
Dodecyl alcohol	25.0	Mineral oil				*
Decyl alcohol	25.0	Mineral oil				*
Propylene glycol diacetate	Neat			*		
Propylene glycol	Neat				*	
Propylene carbonate	Neat				*	

TABLE 2 - continued

Irritancy Ratings of Topical Materials

Agent	Concentration %	Vehicle	Classification			
			Low (0-0.4)	Slight (0.5-1.4)	Moderate (1.5-2.4)	Marked (2.5-4.0)
Vegetable oils						
Safflower oil			*			
Peanut oil			*			
Sesame oil			*			
Olive oil			*			
Linseed oil					*	
Corn oil				*		

Bland Ointments and Creams
_____

Lanolin (hydrous) USP	*		
Petrolatum USP	*		
Carbowax ointment USP	*		
Cold cream USP	*		
Vanishing cream USP	*		
Keri lotion (Westwood)	*		
Lubriderm (Texas Pharmacal)	*		
Noxzema (Noxell)			*
Aquacare cream (Allergan)	*		
Aquacare HP - 10% urea (Allergan)		*	
Nivea cream (Beiersdorf)		*	
Vanishing cream (Pond's)			*
Purpose cream (Johnson & Johnson)			*

TABLE 2 - *continued*

Irritancy Ratings of Topical Materials

Agent	Concentration %	Vehicle	Classification			
			Low (0-0.4)	Slight (0.5-1.4)	Moderate (1.5-2.4)	Marked (2.5-4.0)
Dermassage cream (Colgate-Palmolive)					*	
Zinc oxide ointment USP			*			
Powders						
Talcum powder USP			*			
Kalin NF			*			
Corn starch USP			*			
Zinc oxide powder USP			*			
Magnesium trisilicate powder USP			*			
Titanium dioxide powder			*			

Sodium bicarbonate USP:						
saturated solution	10	Water			*	
powder	10	Talc			*	
powder	neat		*			
Sunscreens						
Amyl-dimethyl -amino benzoic acid	5	Ethanol				*
Octyl-dimethyl -amino benzoic acid	5	Ethanol				*
Glyceryl -amino benzoic acid	5	Ethanol			*	
Surfactants						
Polysorbate-20 (3)	20	Water			*	
Polysorbate-80 (4)	5	Water				*
Polysorbate-85 (5)	5	Water			*	
Amphoteric 2 (6)	20	Water		*		

TABLE 2 - continued

Irritancy Ratings of Topical Materials

Agent	Concentration %	Vehicle	Classification			
			Low (0-0.4)	Slight (0.5-1.4)	Moderate (1.5-2.4)	Marked (2.5-4.0)
Isostearamidopropyl morpholine lactate (7)	2.5	Water		*		
	5.0	Water			*	
	25.0	Water				*
Stearamidopropyl dimethylamine lactate (8)	0.5	Water			*	
	2.5	Water				*
	5.0	Water			*	* (P++)
Triethanolamine	5.0	Ethanol		*		
	10.0	Ethanol				* (P++)
Stearalkonium chloride (9)	1.0	Water		*		
	5.0	Water				*
Octoxynol-9 (10)	1.0	Water		*		
	5.0	Water			*	

Nonoxynol-9 (11)	5.0	Water		*	
	10.0	Water	*		
Laureth-4 (12)	2.0	Water	*		
	10.0	Water			*

Miscellaneous

Crude coal tar	5.0	Hydrophilic ointment	*
Tretinoin cream (13)	0.1		*

Key: P, pustules; Er; Erosions; (1) Irgasan DP 300 (Ciba-Geigy); (2) Hyamine 3500 (Rohn & Haas); (3) Tween 20 (ICI America); (4) Tween 80 (ICI America); (5) Tween 85 (ICI America); (6) Miranol C2M CONC (Miranol); (7) Richamate ISML (Richardson); (8) Richamate 3780 (Richardson); (9) Triton X-400 (Rohn & Haas); (10) Triton X-100 (Rohn & Haas); (11) Tergitol TP 9 (Union Carbide); (12) Brij 30 (ICI America); (13) Retin-A cream (Johnson & Johnson).

145

high SIs. Formaldehyde solution 37% has a high SI of 40 because it is a very toxic substance which damages normal skin
at a low concentration. In contrast, Triton X-100--a very
mild irritant on normal skin--is quite toxic after scarification; this results in a SI of 50. Moreover, there are pecu-
liar substances such as propylene glycol which irritate
scarified and normal skin at about the same concentration.
For the greatest number of substances SIs cannot be determined at all owing to the inability to provoke a reaction on
normal skin.

DOSAGE RESPONSE

As anticipated, the intensity of the reaction increased
with concentration. The plot was roughly linear for the few
substances examined in this way; however, the slope of the
curve was different for different substances varying from
shallow to steep. This adds an additional parameter for comparative assessments. Threshold concentrations may be nearly
identical for two substances when their irritancy potentiali-
ties are really quite different. The surfactants Triton
X-100 and Triton X-400 are a good example. The threshold
concentration for both is about 1%. At 5%, however, Triton
X-100 was still a mild irritant, while Triton X-400 produced
severe reactions. When testing single chemicals rather than
mixtures it will often be valuable to establish the severity
of the response with 2.5 to 5.0 times the threshold concentration.

Triethanolamine, a very common component in cosmetics,
is generally held to be innocuous; this estimate would be
supported by the fact that 10% concentrations produced no
reaction on normal skin. On scarified skin, however, 10%
brought forth a severe inflammatory response. While the
concentration in most creams is generally less than 5.0%,
this may be offset by the fact that these products are used
daily for long periods, not infrequently on damaged skin.
In addition, certain substances may build up on the skin with
repeated use if they have substantive properties. It can be
argued, therefore, that a watchful eye should be placed over
chemicals that cause intense reactions on scarified skin at
5% and 10% concentrations.

SPECIFICITY OF RESPONSE

One requires to know whether the scarification technique
will evoke reactions with substances that from long experience are almost certainly without much irritancy potential.
The advantage of increased sensitivity could be negated by a

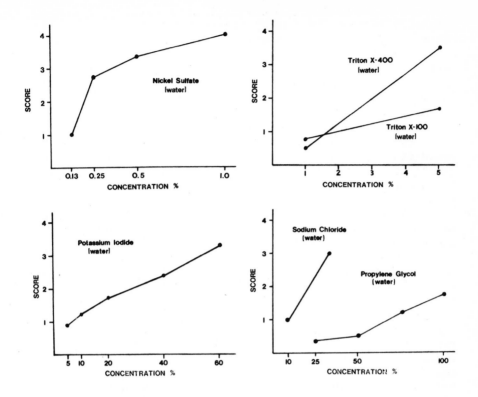

Fig. 5. *Dose-response curves for different substances; the slopes vary greatly but are more or less linear. The steeper slope of Triton X-400 indicates that this substance is more irritating than Triton X-100, though these appear equivalent at 1%.*

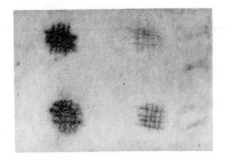

Fig. 6. *Reactions to nickel sulfate in a series of two-fold increases in concentration (0.06, 0.13, 0.25, 0.5). The intensity of the response is sharply dependent on dose.*

greater likelihood of false positive reactions.

We evaluated a great variety of familiar materials, including ones which are generally regarded as very mild
(Table 2). We designated irritancy potential as low when the
mean scores fell between 0 and 0.4, slight when between 0.5
and 1.4, moderate between 1.5 and 2.4, and marked between 2.5
and 4.0.

Reassuringly, bland substances bearing the USP label,
often used as vehicles, produced no reactions; these included
petrolatum, Carbowax ointment, lanolin, cold cream, vanishing
cream, zinc oxide ointment, talcum powder, and corn starch.
Likewise, the common vegetable oils were nonirritating,
although this was not true for linseed oil.

While we have not undertaken a comprehensive evaluation
of proprietary moisturizing creams, it is interesting that
these are not all inert. Pond's Vanishing Cream, Dermassage,
and Purpose might be classified as having mild irritancy
potential. Moreover, the addition of 10 to 20% urea in certain moisturizing creams may confer upon them a slight
potentiality of irritation.

An instructive situation arose in the case of Hydrophilic
Ointment USP. For years we have incorporated various experimental materials in this well-known oil-in-water cream.
Suddenly, we encountered irritant reactions with preparations
that had previously been innocuous. It turned out that we
had purchased Hydrophilic Ointment from a new source (The
Torch Co.). This latter material utilized 1% sodium lauryl
sulfate as the emulsifier according to the specification of
the recent editions of the U.S. Pharmacopea. The Torch
Hydrophilic Ointment caused moderate irritation on scarified
skin and was even somewhat irritating on normal skin.
Bergstresser and Eaglestein had in fact earlier identified
USP Hydrophilic Ointment as an irritant when occlusively
applied for 3 to 5 days on normal skin (9). They showed, as
have we, that sodium lauryl sulfate was the source of irritancy. Though labeled USP the brand of Hydrophilic Ointment
we had used for years (Lannett Co.) was evidently compounded
with a different emulsifier. It caused no reaction on scarified skin. Despite this agreeable feature it is not entitled
to be called USP. In any case, authentic USP Hydrophilic
Ointment is not a good choice for a really bland ointment.

Other illuminating findings were as follows. Gentian
violet, a traditional antimicrobial dye widely used on burns
and superficial skin infections was clearly far from nontoxic.
Indeed, Björnberg and Monacken observed necrotic skin reactions with therapeutic applications of 1% gentian violet
(10). On normal skin, concentrated solutions are harmless, a
strong argument for a more sensitive test method. It is becoming ever more apparent that propylene glycol, extensively

utilized in vehicles, may be irritating in concentrations above 50% (11, 12). This is a curious material which often is no more irritating on scarified than on normal skin. It has too long been taken for granted as "bland."

A surfactant widely heralded as being very mild (Miranol C2M) was, in fact, moderately irritating at a 20% concentration. Dodecyl and decyl alcohols were surprisingly severe irritants at 25% strengths in mineral oils.

A 10% sodium chloride solution produced no reaction, but a 38% aqueous (saturated) solution elicited pustules. It would appear to be the rule that strongly hypertonic solutions are capable of damaging tissue to which they gain access. Pustules are the characteristic reaction to hypertonic solutions of halides (sodium and potassium iodides, chlorides, bromides, and fluorides). It is important to note that pH, despite common beliefs, is of slight significance only. No reactions were observed with 0.1 M buffer solutions (glycine and phosphate buffers) in the pH range 2.0 to 11.0

VEHICLES

It will occasion no surprise that the degree of irritation was strongly dependent on the vehicle. Vehicles chiefly influence irritancy by their effect on release of the test agent and its partitioning into the horny layer.

It is our practice to use aqueous solutions for water-soluble substances and 95% ethanol for lipid-soluble materials that will dissolve in it. For poorly soluble materials we use mineral oil when possible or an appropriate bland cream or oil. One must avoid light mineral oils as these are mild irritants on scarified skin. Irritancy decreases as the flash point increases. It is a little surprising that ethanol was virtually nonirritating; this is doubtlessly attributable to the small volume (100 µl) in the chamber. Other volatile solvents such as chloroform and acetone are highly irritating in chamber exposures.

We briefly evaluated some lipoid-soluble moderate irritants such as hexachlorophene, oleic acid, and lauric acid in different vehicles. Ethanol consistently gave the highest scores, usually followed by mineral oil. Incorporation in creams and particularly ointments produced the lowest scores, as might have been expected. Slow release from thick, oily vehicles doubtless accounts for this. Petrolatum is a typical example. As expected, 5% aluminum chloride was completely nonirritating in petrolatum, moderately irritating in vanishing cream USP, and highly irritating in water.

It is worth noting that powders can be tested directly.

Most common dusting powders like talc, starch, and zinc oxide were, as expected, quite inert. On the other hand, this was not the case for sodium bicarbonate. The neat powder was quite irritating although a 10% solution was not. We were able to show that larger crystals gave more intense reactions. A physical effect is implicated here in addition to hypertonicity. The scarification procedure holds interesting possibilities for testing solid substances which are physically different with regard to the size and shape of crystals.

COMPARISON BETWEEN HYPER- AND HYPOREACTIVE SUBJECTS

No one engaged in extensive testing can fail to observe that individuals differ strikingly in the intensity of inflammatory reactions to irritants. An appreciable proportion of normal persons have integuments which are highly vulnerable to weakly toxic substances. We shall show elsewhere that these hyperreactive subjects generally have more permeable skin, that they react excessively in all body regions, and that their hyperirritability extends virtually to all potential irritants. We are currently evaluating simple procedures for identifying hyperreactors and shall mention here only one. Persons who show a brisk inflammatory reaction on normal forearm skin to a 24 hr chamber exposure of 80% aqueous propylene glycol or 1% sodium lauryl sulfate have hyperirritable skins.

We were greatly interested in finding out whether the scarification test obliterated the intrinsic difference between hyper- and hyporeactive subjects. Scarification tests were performed on these two contrasting groups. The results shown in Table 3 make it clear that the difference between hyper- and hyporeactors is still apparent on scarified skin, though narrower than on normal skin. The difference was most evident at 48 hr often becoming insignificant by 72 hr. This result shows clearly that factors other than the horny layer barrier influence the response to irritants. Hyporeactors evidently have a lower capacity to mount an inflammatory response.

In view of these findings, should one make an effort to select hyperirritable subjects? The answer depends on the degree of discrimination required. For most purposes, preselection is superfluous. It is sufficient to choose young, healthy adults who have no skin problems. On the other hand, the variance is reduced substantially by recruiting only hyperirritable volunteers. As regards susceptibility to irritants our experiences to date have led to the following judgments:

    1. Blacks are less reactive than whites; this is con-

TABLE 3

Comparison between Hypo- and Hyperreactive Individuals (Readings at 48 hr)

Agent	Hyperreactors		Hyporeactors	
	Scarified	Normal skin	Scarified	Normal skin
Propylene glycol (neat)	1.2	1.2	0.2	0.2
Vanishing cream (Pond's)	1.4	1.2	0.3	0.2
0.1% Tretinoin cream (J&J)	2.2	0.6	1.4	0
5% Decyl alcohol (mineral oil)	2.2	1.0	1.6	0
5% Triton X-100 (water	2.0	0	1.2	0
30% Urea (water)	2.4	0	0.8	0
5% Aluminum chloride (water)	3.2	0	2.4	0
10% Potassium iodide (water)	2.2	0	1.0	0

sistent with the findings of Weigand and Gaylor, who showed
that the stratum corneum of blacks is a more effective
barrier to dinitrochlorobenzene (13).

2.   Caucasoids of light complexion who sunburn easily
and tan easily are more susceptible than darker, Mediter-
ranean types.   Light complexion alone is, however, not
reliable without the sunburning history and evidence of
Celtic origin.

3.   There is a hint, but no more, that females may be
slightly more vulnerable.

TIME RELATIONSHIPS

A single reading after 72 hr of exposure is usually quite
sufficient for appraising irritancy potential.   Daily readings, on the other hand, give additional information and may
furnish a greater degree of discrimination.

With most mild irritants, there is no reaction at 24 hr,
a variable one at 48 hr, and definite responses by 72 hr.
Despite some exceptions, longer exposures do not confer a
proportionate promotion of sensitivity.   The corresponding
increase in labor, time, and cost is not warranted.   It may
on occasion be useful to make another reading at 96 hr a day
after removing the chamber.

With stronger irritants, daily scoring may show interesting contrasts.   Two materials may produce identically mild
reactions on the first day.   For one material, further exposures may result in a sharp increase in the intensity of
the reaction, accompanied by vivid expressions such as blis-
ters or erosions, while for the other, the reaction may have
increased only modestly by the end of three days.   For strong
irritants, 1 day exposures may be sufficient.   For the great
majority of materials of dermatologic and cosmetic interest
we use the full 3 day exposure period, even when reactions
are evident earlier.   This provides a chance to follow the
evolution of the response and to note special changes such
as pustules.

DISCUSSION

We would call attention to the qualifying adverb which
we have assiduously employed throughout this work, namely
potentially irritating.   The ratings are purely relative and
apply only to this testing system.   We do not suppose that
the scores can be used with any degree of confidence to predict what the level of irritation will be in actual use.
Scarification and continuous exposure in a chamber are a far

cry from customary uses.

The actual hazard can only be roughly estimated and will be dependent on frequency of use (including misuse), body region, normalcy of skin, geography (tropics versus temperate regions), season, and other factors. One certainly does not automatically exclude materials with even moderate irritating scores if these possess other highly desirable features. In that case, one strategy is to proceed to a usage test in which the product is applied in the intended way two to three times more often. The scarification test may be altogether inappropriate for some materials, viz., those in which the active ingredients are dissolved in irritating, volatile solvents, unless the solvent is evaporated first. On the other hand, low scores (0.5) are a guarantee of mildness no matter how the product may be used.

To add to the manifest benefits of the savings in cost, time, and effort we would emphasize the increase in sensitivity and reproducibility provided by the scarification method. One can get the same results time after time to a degree not possible with patch tests. Also, special cutaneous displays such as pustules, vesicles, and erosions occur more rapidly with scarification. We find, in addition, that seasonal effects are less pronounced with the scarification technique. Irritant responses characteristically diminish in summer; this change is evidently muted by scarification.

For definitive testing we select hyperirritable subjects based on a sharp reaction to a 24 hr exposure to 80% propylene glycol or 1% sodium lauryl sulfate. Ten young adult Caucasoids constitute a test panel for routine testing.

What are the hazards of scarification? Infection is exceedingly rare; we do not recall a clear-cut instance in all our experience though the possibility cannot be ruled out. Scarification, the name notwithstanding, leaves no scars. Severe inflammatory responses may produce permanent change but are limited to experimental demonstrations. Ordinarily one will not be evaluating highly irritating materials. We have developed this method mainly to provide enhanced sensitivity for the appraisal of mild irritants.

ACKNOWLEDGMENTS

We would like to thank Mrs. T. Kwong, Mrs. S. Duncan, and Miss C. Cass for their expert assistance.

REFERENCES

1. Kligman, A. M., and Wooding, W. M. (1967). A method for the measurement and evaluation of irritants in human skin. *J. Invest. Dermatol. 49*:78.
2. Lanman, B. M., Elvers, W. B., and Howard, C. S. (1968). The role of human patch testing in a product development program. In *Proceedings, Joint Conference on Cosmetic Sciences*, pp. 135-145. Washington, D. C., The Toilet Goods Association.
3. Finkelstein, P., Laden, K., and Mizchowski, W. (1963). New methods for evaluating cosmetic irritancy. *J. Invest. Dermatol. 40*:11.
4. Pirilä, V. (1975). Chamber test versus patch test for epicutaneous testing. *Contact Dermatitis 1*:48.
5. Magnusson, B., and Hersle, K. (1965). Patch-test methods. II. Regional variations of patch test responses. *Acta Derm.-Venereol. 45*:257.
6. Blank, I. A., Jones, J. L., and Gould, E. (1958). A study of the penetration of aluminum salts into excised human skin. *Cosmet. J. 29*:32.
7. Uehara, M., Takahashi, C., and Ofuji, S. (1975). Pustular patch test reactions in atopic dermatitis. *Arch. Dermatol. 111*:1154.
8. Mezei, M. (1975). Effect of polysorbate 85 on human skin. *J. Invest. Dermatol. 64*:165.
9. Bergstresser, P. R., and Eaglestein, W. H. (1975). Irritation by hydrophilic ointment under occlusion. *Arch. Dermatol. 108*:218.
10. Björnberg, A., and Monacken, H. (1971). Necrotic skin reactions caused by 1% gentian violet and brilliant green. *Acta Derm.-Venereol. 52*:56.
11. Warshaw, T. G., and Hermann, F. (1952). Studies of skin reactions to propylene glycol. *J. Invest. Dermatol. 19*:423.
12. Shore, R. N., and Shelley, W. B. (1974). Contact dermatitis from stearyl alcohol and propylene glycol in fluocinonide cream. *Arch. Dermatol. 109*:397.
13. Weigand, D. A., Gaylor, J. R. (1974). Irritant reaction in negro and caucasian skin. *South. Med. J. 67*:548.

Prediction of Skin Irritancy and Sensitizing Potential by Testing with Animals and Man

John F. Griffith and Edwin V. Buehler

Ivorydale Technical Center and Miami Valley Laboratories
The Procter and Gamble Company
Cincinnati, Ohio

The possibility that consumers may develop irritant or allergic skin reactions is an important consideration in the development of new chemicals or products. The certainty with which that possibility can be predicted or minimized may help identify the marketing risk.

In the evaluation of the irritant and sensitizing effects of chemicals on the skin, there is the advantage of the possibility of performing tests with human subjects and thus avoiding some of the uncertainties associated with interpretation of animal responses. This is not to say that animal tests should be omitted, for they should not be, at least not with new or unknown materials. Just how animal and human tests relate to one another in making safety predictions in skin irritation and sensitization is our subject for discussion. Our presentation will be limited to, first, a comparison of primary irritant effects obtained by patch testing guinea pigs, rabbits, and humans, and second, a comparison of some results of testing for contact sensitization in guinea pigs and humans.

PRIMARY IRRITANT EVALUATION

Since Draize *et al.*(1) described their rabbit ptach test for primary irritation in 1944, that method has become a

common animal test procedure used by most testing laboratories. It has also been adopted, with various modifications, by government agencies such as the Consumer Product
Safety Commission, Food and Drug Administration, Environmental Protection Agency, and Department of Transportation.
This is not to say that the rabbit has exclusive jurisdiction,
for other animal species, especially the guinea pig, are
favored in some laboratories and their value is recognized
(2); it is just that the "Draize" test with the rabbit is
the most standardized.

COMPARISON OF ANIMAL AND HUMAN RESPONSES

Recent modifications of the Draize primary irritation
test, one adopted (3) and one proposed (4), have been made
with the objective of more nearly simulating actual human
exposure to substances that are likely to be removed from
the skin shortly after exposure than does the method presently used (5). Nixon *et al.* (6), in our laboratories,
have used this proposed procedure with a number of chemicals
and products on rabbits, guinea pigs, and human volunteers.
Fifteen household products and nine chemicals covering a
range from nonirritating to corrosive were patch tested by
this method. Intact and abraded skin was used, except that
some of the most irritating substances were not tested on
either abraded or normal human skin.

Patches were applied for 4 hr and any reactions at
the test sites were scored separately for erythema and
edma (1) after 4, 24, and 48 hours. Primary irritation
indices were calculated from the average of scores for intact and abraded sites. For each species, the result was
classified as negligible, slight, moderate, severe, or corrosive. A corrosive effect was recorded if substantial
tissue destruction or irreversible effects (e.g., scarring)
were seen on intact skin, but not on abraded skin. Criteria
for evaluating rabbit and guinea pig skin reactions were
those of Draize (7). Different and more stringent ranges
were used for human skin reactions on the basis of other
experience with human skin responses and our judgment as to
what these responses should be called. Table 1 compares
the ranges of scores and criteria for animal and human responses. For this purpose "negligible" and "slight" reactions are collectively referred to as "weak," and "severe"
is called "strong."

The effects of ten chemicals tested on human, guinea pig,
and rabbit skin are shown in Table 2. The mean scores given
are those for intact skin, and they are arranged in

TABLE 1

PRIMARY IRRITANT RESPONSE CATEGORIES

	Mean Score	
	Human	Rabbit/G. Pig
Weak	0 - 1.4	0 - 1.9
Moderate	1.5 - 2.4	2.0 - 4.9
Strong	2.5 - 8.0	5.0 - 8.0
Corrosive	Severe tissue destruction or irreversible change	

TABLE 2

Skin Responses to Chemicals (4 hr Patch Test)

	Mean score (intact skin)		
Material	Human	Guinea Pig	Rabbit
Isopropyl alcohol, 100%	0.0	0.0	0.0
Table salt, 50%	0.0	0.0	0.0
Sodium tripolyphosphate, 50%	0.0	0.0	0.0
Sodium carbonate, 50%	0.0	0.0	0.0
Sulfuric acid, 10%	0.2	0.0	0.0
Sodium lauryl sulfate, 50%	0.6	0.0	1.6
Acetic acid, 10%	1.0	0.0	0.0
C_8 - C_{10} fatty acid, 100%	2.3	0.1	4.4
Sodium metasilicate, 50%	--	1.7	C[a]
Potassium hydroxide, 10%	--	C	C

[a]C = corrosive.

order of increasing irritancy to human skin. Sodium metasilicate and potassium hydroxide are known to be potentially corrosive and were therefore not tested on humans. It can be seen that the animal results were accurately predictive for the first five chemicals--those that are essentially nonirritating to human skin. For sodium lauryl sulfate and C_8-C_{10} fatty acid, weakly and moderately irritating respectively, guinea pig skin was less responsive and rabbit skin was more responsive. The presumably corrosive metasilicate and potassium hydroxide were found to be so on rabbit skin, but only the latter was corrosive to guinea pig skin.

Of the household products (Table 3), four laundry detergents were all classified as weakly irritant, though rabbit responses were somewhat more intense than those seen with humans or guinea pigs. These and the next five products gave little or no response in humans or guinea pigs. Though the guinea pig results were generally predictive of the human results, rabbit responses to the soap, the liquid detergent, and the cleaner would incorrectly place these products in the next higher, or moderate irritant category. Of the last five products, two (shampoo, pine oil cleaner) were weakly irritant, one (ammonia) was moderately irritating, and two (metasilicate detergent and bleach) were strongly irritating to human skin. Neither the guinea pig nor the rabbit skin would have predicted any of these responses correctly on the basis of absolute scores. Three of the rabbit results erred on the high side and two on the low side; the opposite was true for the guinea pig.

The overall accuracy of predictions from animal results is summarized in Table 4. By the criteria defined in Table 1, rabbit and guinea pig skin gave 16 "correct" results in 24 trials on intact skin. Both species tended to err on the high side with "weak" irritants; the guinea pig was more often on the low side with "moderate" or stronger irritants.

Though we have emphasized only the data from tests on intact skin, the situation was not improved by using abraded skin; rather it was made worse. Of 21 materials for which comparisons were carried out with abraded skin (Table 5), correct classification was obtained in nine instances by the guinea pig test. As with intact skin, errors in evaluating irritancy were on the high side with both species for weak materials and on the low side with the guinea pig for moderate to corrosive materials. Furthermore, and more importantly, with none of 19 materials actually tested on abraded human skin was there an average response that would be classified differently from the average response to the same material on intact skin.

TABLE 3

Skin Responses to Household Products

Material	Mean Score (intact skin)		
	Human	Guinea Pig	Rabbit
Detergent granules:			
Low carbonate, 50%	0.0	0.1	0.7
High carbonate, 50%	0.0	0.0	0.9
Enzyme, 50%	0.0	0.0	1.3
Phosphate, 50%	0.0	0.2	1.2
Coconut oil soap, 50%	0.0	0.3	2.5
Antiperspirant, 100%	0.1	0.0	0.0
Liquid detergent, 100%	0.1	0.8	2.4
Lemon juice, 100%	0.2	0.0	0.0
Liquid cleaner, 100%	0.2	0.3	3.0
Liquid shampoo, 100%	0.9	2.1	3.7
Pine oil cleaner, 100%	1.0	2.5	3.6
Household ammonia, 100%	1.5	0.0	1.4
Metasilicate-carbonate detergent, 50%	3.0	0.0	C[a]
Hypochlorite bleach, 100%	3.9	0.3	1.0

[a] C = corrosive.

TABLE 4

Human vs. Animal Test Result (24 Materials; Intact Skin)

	Weak	Moderate	Strong	Corrosive
Guinea pig:				
Less		2	2	1
Same	16			
More	2			1
Rabbit:				
Less		1	1	
Same	13	1		2
More	5		1	

TABLE 5

Human vs. Animal Test Result (21 Materials; Abraded Skin)

	Weak	Moderate	Strong	Corrosive
Guinea pig:				
Less		2	1	1
Same	13			1
More	3			
Rabbit:				
Less		2		
Same	7			2
More	9		1	

SUMMARY

Based on evaluations of primary irritations by the 4 hr patch test, several conclusions can be reached regarding the response obtained in different species, the value of using abraded skin, and the significance of responses obtained with a semiocclusive patch test.

1. Rabbit skin reacts somewhat more severely than guinea pig or human skin to primary irritants. This could be *partly* compensated for by establishing different score evaluation criteria for each species and by carrying out more extensive comparative studies with humans.

2. Disagreements of animal with human results almost always involved stronger reactions of animals to weak irritants; in contrast, the guinea pig showed weaker reactions to strong irritants. This makes the use of standard irritant materials of similar chemical and physical properties and known human irritancy an important adjunct to any irritancy evaluation that uses *only* animal tests. By using such controls in comparative studies it should be possible to predict whether a material is more or less irritating to human skin than the control.

3. For weak irritants guinea pig skin reactions are more predictive of human response than rabbit skin reactions. From these data and our experience with this species in sensitization testing, we believe that guinea pig skin is more tolerant of strong irritants and corrosive materials than is human skin. For the rabbit, the opposite is true, so that the responses of this species to strong irritants seem to be more predictive of human responses. This suggests that the best model may be dependent on the type of material to be tested. Furthermore, if the composition and probable irritancy of the material are unknown, it would be useful to make some preliminary evaluation of its chemical and physical characteristics for use in the selection of a suitable comparative irritant standard.

4. Irritancy data from tests on abraded skin lead to substantially the same classification of materials as data from intact skin tests, or from averages of the two (i.e., the Draize Primary Irritation Index). As abraded skin increases animal requirements, expense and complexity of tests, a requirement for such testing seems counterproductive. More useful data could be obtained by expending the effort on tests with a second species.

5. Though a 4 hr semiocclusive patch test seems a more realistic exposure than one of 24 hr for evaluating many types of household products, usage conditions or special properties of the material could call for longer or shorter exposures, or for tests of other than full-strength product.

Indeed, the time of exposure that will produce a definite
irritant end point might be a preferable alternative to the
use of a single exposure duration in quantifying the irritant potential of a material. It stands to reason that a
material that will produce frank skin irritation on contact
of a few minutes could be more hazardous than one that takes
several hours to evoke the same response.

SENSITIZATION POTENTIAL

    After primary irritation, the next important considera-
tion in the cutaneous safety evaluation of a consumer product or its ingredients is the potential for causing contact
sensitization, or more specifically, delayed contact hypersensitivity. As this is an allergic phenomenon that can
result in a permanent alteration of a person's responsiveness to an agent and can evoke a protracted dermatitis if
contact with that agent occurs, manufacturers wish to avoid
selling products that will sensitize. Thus, the screening
of chemicals and products for sensitization potential is an
essential part of any consumer product development program.
    Although it is possible to work directly with human sub-
jects in testing for sensitization, it is prudent to screen
new substances first by testing with animals. For this
purpose, the albino guinea pig is the species of choice, as
it will respond well to most strong sensitizers (8). The
protocol used in our laboratories is a closed, i.e., occlusive, repeated patch test that was developed by one of us (8)
to mimic the familiar human repeated insult patch test of
Shelanski and Shelanski (9). The technique takes advantage
of the ability of guinea pig skin to tolerate rather high
concentrations of topically applied chemicals without excessive primary irritation. At the same time it utilizes
the practical and appropriate percutaneous route of absorption so that the potential hapten may have the contact
with the protein of the epidermis that is necessary for
complete antigen formation. We recognize that this procedure allows the epidermis to act as a barrier to some
materials that might sensitize at lower levels if introduced systemically, but we believe that a practical screening technique should not bypass the important biological
barrier of the epidermis as is the case with the various
intradermal techniques.

EVALUATIONS OF THE CLOSED PATCH TEST

    The guinea pig closed patch test was employed, and test
compound was applied to the skin for a 6 hr treatment period

once each week for 3 successive weeks. There were 15 to 20
animals in each treatment group and the test substance was
applied at as high a concentration as possible that would
not cause excessive irritation. This induction series was
followed in 2 weeks by dual 6 hr challenge patches on the
depilated flanks of each animal. An equal number of previously untreated animals was challenged as a control. A
third group was carried through the entire test as a vehicle
control for whatever solvent or suspending agent was used
with the test material. Each patch site was graded for
erythema 24 and 48 hr after removal of the patches. The significance of reactions in the test material group was then
evaluated relative to any reactions seen in the two control
groups, so that either a greater incidence or a greater intensity of reactions relative to the controls was considered to be indicative of sensitization.

This closed patch test procedure has been compared with
other techniques for inducing contact sensitization in
guinea pigs. In one experiment (8) animals were exposed by
patch, intradermal injection, and by topical application of
1-chloro-2,4-dinitrobenzene (dinitrochlorobenzene, DNCB).
The closed patch gave the highest incidence of sensitization
(Table 6), and there was less interference from primary irritation as the test could be conducted with a lower concentration of DNCB. Some comparisons of the incidence of sensitization using equal concentration of materials administered
by closed patch or intradermal injection are shown in Table
7. Tetrachlorosalicylanilide, *p*-phenylenediamine, thiogly-
cerol, and monobenzyl ether of hydroquinone did not induce
sensitization by the intradermal route but did by epicutaneous exposure under a closed patch. More comparable but
lower rates of sensitization resulted with formalin and
potassium chromate. Attempts at sensitization with salts of
mercury, cobalt, and nickel were unsuccessful by either
technique.

More recently, one of our colleagues, Dr. H. L. Ritz
(personal communication), has compared the rates of sensitization to 1-alkenyl-1,3-sultones using an epicutaneous
route of spplication (i.e., the closed patch) with that of a
single intradermal injection in Freund's complete adjuvant
(Table 8). The unsaturated sultones are examples of a recently characterized class of potent human sensitizers (11),
and they were apparently responsible for an epidemic of
contact dermatitis that occurred in Norway in 1966 when the
sultones were present as a contaminant in a dishwashing
detergent (12, 13, 14).

Table 8 shows the responses to epicutaneous challenges
in the guinea pig with different amounts of two unsaturated
sultones having 12 and 16 carbon atoms (H. L. Ritz,

TABLE 6

Effectiveness of Different Methods of Sensitization with Dinotrochlorobenzene in the Guinea Pig

	Incidence (%)
Closed patch:	
0.05% DNCB	100
0.01% DNCB	40–50
Intradermal injection:	
0.25% DNCB	30
0.05% DNCB	0
Topical application:	
0.5% DNCB	70
0.1% DNCB	0

unpublished observations). These followed either intradermal induction with 7.1, 71, or 710 nanomoles or epicutaneous induction with 71, 710, or 7100 nanomoles of sensitizer. The table illustrates that, though the use of Freund's adjuvant lessens the amount of sultone required to induce sensitization, the technique has, more importantly, altered the *relative* sensitization potential of the C_{12} versus the C_{16} sultone, as compared with the epicutaneous results. This suggests that caution must be exercised in assigning relative sensitizing activity to topical agents that are tested intradermally with Freund's complete adjuvant. This may be a more important practical consideration than the relative sensitivity of the two methods when using one or the other as a screening test prior to a human sensitization test. As most new or unknown materials should be screened at concentrations as high as can be reasonably tolerated, either method may be expected to screen out potentially strong sensitizers to human skin, but the technique relying on induction by percutaneous absorption should reflect more accurately the importance of the epidermal barrier in anticipated topical usage.

TABLE 7

Epicutaneous vs. Intradermal Testing for Sensitization

Compound	Incidence[a]	
	Patch	I.D.
p-Phenylenediamine HCl, 2%	10/10	0/10
Tetrachlorosalicylanilide, 1%	8/10	0/10
Thioglycerol, 14%	6/10	0/10
Monobenzyl ether of hydroquinone, 5%	3/5	0/10
Formalin, 5%	3/10	1/10
Potassium chromate, 1%	1/10	1/10

[a]Number of guinea pigs sensitized/number tested.

The human sensitization test that we use is a modification of the method of Shelanski and Shelanski (9), and it has been described in detail in a previous symposium sponsored by these two societies (15). Solutions of materials are applied to cotton felt pads placed on the dorsal skin of the upper arm and covered by a completely occlusive adhesive backing. These patches, which are left on the skin for 24 hr, are applied 3 days a week (Monday, Wednesday, and Friday) for 3 weeks. Usually it is convenient to test four materials simultaneously. Successive applications are to the same site, unless irritation necessitates relocation. Following this induction series, there is a 2 week period during which no patches are applied. At the beginning of the 6th week, each subject is challenged with the test materials at the same sites as used for induction and at fresh sites on the opposite arm. The challenge patches are removed at 24 hr and any responses are graded immediately and at 48 and 96 hr. Reactions suggestive of sensitization are confirmed by a second challenge 2 months after the first challenge.

Concentrations of materials used in the procedure are based on the highest concentration expected in use or in other reasonably anticipated exposure. It can be full strength if prolonged contact with undiluted product is

TABLE 8

Sensitization with 1-Alkenyl-1,3-Sultones

Compound	Challenge, nmole	Response to sensitization dose, nmole[a]					
		Intradermal			Epicutaneous		
		7.1	71	710	71	710	7100
C_{12}	200	15/15	14/14	11/15	9/15	13/15	13/14
	20	15/15	11/14	7/15	4/15	8/15	10/14
	2	12/15	7/14	1/15	2/15	6/15	9/14
C_{16}	200	15/15	15/15	11/15	0/14	1/15	6/15
	20	14/15	13/15	0/15	0/14	0/15	1/15
	2	6/15	3/15	0/15	0/14	0/15	1/15

[a] Number sensitized/number tested.

expected. If such exposure results in more than moderate
primary irritation, test concentrations are reduced to a
tolerable level. In our experience, primary irritation has
not been a necessary prerequisite for the induction of delayed contact hypersensitivity. Indeed, the concept of
"maximizing" exposure to a potential allergen by also ex-
posing the skin to a strong irritant, as advanced by Kligman
(16), complicates any practical interpretation of observed
reactions, as this procedure is predicated on the idea that
most chemicals have some potential for sensitization that
could better be compared if the cutaneous barrier is removed
as an interfering variable.

PREDICTABILITY OF SENSITIZATION TESTS

We believe that in order to be a reliable predictive
tool a sensitization test should provide at least as much or
more intense exposure to a product or material than the consumer would be expected to experience in normal use. But we
also believe that the human test exposure should bear some
practical relationship to the actual usage exposure. Thus,
the simple expedient of increasing the concentration of a
single component of a product may alter the chemical or
physical environment in a formulation to the point that the
test is not realistic. Even if exaggeration of concentration is not feasible, other features of the patch test can
exaggerate the intensity of exposure: (a) the material may
be held in contact with the skin longer than in a usage situation, (b) the frequency of application may be greater, and
(c) occlusion can be expected to increase penetration. However, the overall degree of exaggeration provided in a test
cannot be calculated with any certainty, as several different kinds of variables are in operation at the same time.
One way in which a sensitization test obviously cannot
exaggerate real-life exposure is in the number of subjects
involved. The exposure through marketing is potentially
many millions, but skin patch tests are customarily performed on only 100-200 people before a product is marketed.
The statistical analysis made by Henderson and Riley (17)
of the reliance that can be placed on negative patch test
results from panels of various sizes is often mentioned in
this context. This analysis depended on the assumptions
that the test panel is a representative sample of the population and that the patch-test procedure will detect materials that will truly produce allergic reactions. However,
the analysis did not deal with the quantitative relationships and variations between exposures under patch-test conditions and those under normal use. Thus, the statistical
projections depend on identical conditions for testing and

use, conditions that are probably not realized in most situations.

The Henderson and Riley analysis shows that if there are no positive reactions to a product in a test panel of 100 subjects the rate of positive reactions in the general population is not likely to exceed 2.9% at the 95% level of confidence. A 2.9% level of sensitization in the general populations would obviously be intolerable for a consumer product. This suggests that more people should be patch tested to improve the reliability of positive reactions, but even if there are no reactions on testing 1,000 people, the likelihood of positive reactions in the population is reduced only to 0.3%. This is still not an acceptable figure, for it suggests that if 1/20 the total U.S. population, or approximately 10 million, were exposed to the product, 30,000 might be expected to become allergic to it. It is quite obvious from the low numbers of actual allergic responses to most products that nothing approaching tens of thousands of allergic reactions occur as would be predicted by this analysis.

How then does one place any reliance on "zero incidence" data from sensitization tests involving 100 people, more or less, when preparing to market a new product? One answer is to have reliable test methods and to use them in a way that truly tests the product or chemical. If we know that a test will detect a sensitizer that has caused actual clinical sensitization we can then be more confident in basing decisions on positive or negative data from that test. As we have shown, the guinea pig closed patch test is capable of detecting moderate to strong sensitizers. How does it compare, then, with the human repeated insult patch test in this ability, or in the ability of the human test to detect moderate and weak sensitizers? Table 9 lists six materials which we have tested by both methods. In most cases, concentrations used in the guinea pig test were higher than in the human test, and vehicles were not necessarily the same.

With reference to Table 9 it should be noted that benzoyl peroxide preparations used in treatment of acne have occasionally resulted in contact sensitivity (18, 19, 20). It was also found by patch testing (21) that an experimental acne preparation of 10% benzoyl peroxide and 1% sulfur suspended in polyethylene glycol was equally sensitizing to guinea pigs and humans.

Though it is generally notorious as a photosensitizer, tetrachlorosalicylanilide (TCSA) is less well known as a contact sensitizer. We detected the sensitizing action in human tests (0.01 to 0.05% in aqueous detergent solution) before our guinea pig test was developed. Later confirmation in guinea pigs was done with a 1% ethanol solution of TCSA (Table 9).

TABLE 9

Rate of Sensitization in Guinea Pigs and Humans *(Number Sensitized/Number Exposed)*

	Guinea pig		Human	
	Conc., %	Rate	Conc., %	Rate
Benzoyl peroxide/sulfur	10	8/19	10	28/69
Tetrachlorosalicylanilide	1.0	8/10	0.05	31/163
Dithio quaternary ammonium compound	1.0	19/19	0.2	8/73
Sulfonyl compound	0.5	0.20	0.5	5/66
Hydroxylamine sulfate	0.2	0/20	0.05	3/76
1-(3-Chlorophenyl)-3-phenyl-2-pyrazoline	1.0	0/20	0.05	2/68

Two experimental antimicrobial agents, one a dithio-quaternary ammonium compound and the other a sulfonyl compound, were moderate sensitizers in human testing, but guinea pig studies gave divergent results. The quaternary ammonium compound was a strong sensitizer in guinea pigs at 1% in ethanol, but less potent in humans at 0.2% in aqueous surfactant. The sulfonyl compound, when tested at 0.5% in an antiperspirant in both animal and human tests, induced no reactions in guinea pigs, compared to 7% positive reactions in humans (Table 9).

Hydroxylamine sulfate did not sensitize guinea pigs at 15% in surfactant solution, but sensitized 3 of 76 human subjects at 0.05% in a detergent solution (Table 9).

Finally, a fluorescent whitening agent, 1-(3-chloro-phenyl)-3-phenyl-2-pyrazoline, did not sensitize guinea pigs when applied at 1% in ethanol, but caused sensitization in human subjects at 0.05% in aqueous detergent solution (22). On this basis we rejected it, though it has been used by others abroad. Osmundsen (23) has attributed several cases of dermatitis in Denmark to this material.

An interesting example of the ability of these patch-test techniques to detect what must surely be considered a weak (or rare) sensitizer is provided by ethanol. We have used ethanol in various concentrations and in different combinations as a vehicle. Occasionally spurious results have occurred with both guinea pigs and humans that have been explainable only as hypersensitivity to ethanol. As these reactions were complicated by the presence of other materials, e.g., surfactants, experiments were performed to see if sensitization to pure ethanol could be induced in the absence of all other materials (except water, used as a diluent) (24). Guinea pigs were treated, using the standard closed patch procedure, with 80% ethanol, but no reactions were seen following a single challenge. A second challenge 9 days after the first resulted in an incidence of 12 reactions in the 18 treated animals, as compared with none in control animals.

Ninety-three human subjects were also tested, using 50% ethanol for induction. At the first challenge, 15 subjects appeared possibly to be sensitized. Fourteen were rechallenged after 2 months with several concentrations of ethanol, with the results shown in Table 10, which shows the lowest concentration to which they reacted (6.25% was also the lowest concentration tested). These reactions were by no means equivocal, being clearly vesicular. Since they were patch tested, the sensitized subjects have undoubtedly had wide exposure to ethanol, but none has, as yet, reported any dermatological problems to us. On the other hand, we are avoiding further use of high concentrations of ethanol as a test vehicle in human studies.

TABLE 10

Human Sensitization with 50% Ethanol

Subjects tested	93
Subjects possibly sensitized	15
Sensitization confirmed:	
50% ethanol	6
25% ethanol	4
12.5% ethanol	2
6.25% ethanol	2

SUMMARY

We have presented evidence that:

1. The closed patch test in the guinea pig provides a sensitive technique for detecting many strong contact sensitizers as well as some moderate and weak ones so that human exposure to such materials can be minimized.
2. Epicutaneous induction can result in a different order of potency of sensitizers than intradermal induction using Fruend's complete adjuvant, and this may have important implications regarding practical exposures to topical agents.
3. The human repeated-insult patch test provides additional sensitivity over that of the guinea pig closed patch test, making it an effective screening procedure in the safety evaluation of topical agents.

REFERENCES

1. Draize, J. H., Woodward, G., and Calvery, H. O. (1944). Methods for the study of irritation and toxicity of substances applied topically to skin and mucous membranes. *J. Pharmacol. Exp. Ther. 82*:377.
2. Lehman, A. J., Fassett, D. W., Gerarde, H. W., Stokinger, H. E., and Zapp, J. Q. (1964). *Principles and Procedures for Evaluating the Toxicity of Household Substances*, p. 9. Washington, D.C., National Academy

of Sciences-National Research Council.

3. Code of Federal Regulations (1975). Title 49, Part 173.240, National Archives of the United States, Washington, D.C.

4. Edwards, C. C. (1972). Hazardous substances. Proposed revision of test for primary skin irritants. *Fed. Regist.* *37*:27635.

5. Code of Federal Regulations (1973). Title 16, Part 1500.41, National Archives of the United States, Washington, D.C.

6. Nixon, G. A., Tyson, C. A., and Wertz, W. C. (1975). Interspecies comparisons of skin irritancy. *Toxicol. Appl. Pharmacol.* *31*:481.

7. Draize, J. H. (1959). Dermal Toxicity. In *Appraisal of Chemicals in Foods, Drugs and Cosmetics*, pp. 46-48. Austin, Tex., Assoc. Food and Drug Officials of the U.S.

8. Buehler, E. V. (1965). Delayed contact hypersensitivity in the guinea pig. *Arch. Dermatol.* *91*:171.

9. Shelanski, H. A., and Shelanski, M. V. (1953). A new technique of human patch tests. *Proc. Sci. Sect. Toilet Goods Assoc.* *19*:46.

10. Landsteiner, K., and Jacobs, J. (1935). Studies on sensitization of animals with simple chemical compounds. *J. Exp. Med.* *61*:643.

11. Ritz, H. L., Connor, D. S., and Sauter, E. D. (1975). Contact sensitization of guinea pigs with unsaturated and halogenated sultones. *Contact Dermatitis* *1*:349.

12. Magnusson, B., and Gilje, O. (1973). Allergic contact dermatitis from a dishwashing liquid containing lauryl ether sulfate. *Acta Derm.-Venereol.* *53*:136.

13. Walker, A. P., Ashforth, G. K., Davies, R. E., Newmann, E. A., and Ritz, H. L. (1973). Some characteristics of the sensitizer in alkyl ethoxy sulphate. *Acta Derm.- Venereol.* *53*:141.

14. Connor, D. S., Ritz. H. L., Ampulski, R. S., Kowollik, H. G., Lim, P., Thomas, D. W., and Parkhurst, R. (1975). Identification of certain sultones as the sensitizers in an alkyl ethoxy sulfate. *Fette, Seifen, Anstrichm.* *77*:25.

15. Griffith, J. F. (1969). Predictive and diagnostic testing for contact sensitization. *Toxicol. Appl. Pharmacol. Suppl.* *3*, p. 90.

16. Kligman, A. M. (1966). The identification of contact allergens by human assay. III. The maximization test: A procedure for screening and rating contact sensitizers. *J. Invest. Dermatol.* *47*:393.

17. Henderson, C. R., and Riley, E. C. (1945). Certain statistical considerations in patch testing. *J. Invest. Dermatol.* *6*:227.

18. Pace, W. E. (1965). A benzoyl peroxide-sulfur cream
     for acne vulgaris. *Can. Med. Assoc. J. 93*:252.
19. Vasarinsh, P. (1968). Benzoyl peroxide-sulfur lotions
     - a histological study. *Arch. Dermatol. 98*:183.
20. Eaglestein, W. H. (1968). Allergic contact dermatitis
     to benzoyl peroxide. *Arch. Dermatol. 97*:527.
21. Poole, R. L., Griffith, J. F., and Mac Millan, F. S. K.
     (1970). Experimental contact sensitization with
     benzoyl peroxide. *Arch. Dermatol. 102*:635.
22. Griffith, J. F. (1973). Fluorescent whitening agents.
     Tests for sensitizing potential. *Arch. Dermatol. 107*:
     728.
23. Osmundsen, P. E. (1969). Contact dermatitis due to an
     optical whitener in washing powders. *Br. J. Dermatol.
     81*:799.
24. Stotts, J., and Ritz., H. L. (1976). Personal communi-
     cation.

In Vitro Experimental Approaches
to Detection of Sensitive Agents*

Albert E. Munson, Beverly A. Barrett, and Joseph F. Borzelleca
Department of Pharmacology and the Cancer Center
Medical College of Virginia
Virginia Commonwealth University
Richmond, Virginia

The studies in this report represent preliminary experiments in a long-range program aimed at developing *in vitro* methods for detection of agents which have potential for producing allergic reactions. Being made cognizant of the need for *in vitro* methods for the prediction of sensitization we hypothesized that agents which elicit a sensitization mediated by the immune system should stimulate a clone of immunocompetent cells to leave the G-1 phase of the cell cycle, enter into DNA synthesis phase, and then proliferate. If they do enter into the act of cycling we propose that detection should be possible by measuring increased macromolecular synthesis, that is, increase in DNA synthesis, RNA synthesis, or protein synthesis. Some of the constraints in this hypothesis are as follows. (i) For any given antigen, the number of lymphoid cells which will respond is very small and may be undetectable by conventional culturing techniques. (ii) Other events must precede the interaction with immunocompetent cells. In the case of cutaneous sensitizing agents, the binding to the skin protein and the processing by macrophage must occur prior to turning on the lymphocyte. (iii) The biochemical events which occur at the level of the

*This investigation was supported by U.S. Public Health Service Research Grants CA 17551, DA 01312, and R 804290010.

175

lymphocyte may not express themselves at the level of the skin. Cutaneous reactions are usually Type I or Type II reactions, that is, the reaction is mediated by IgE, which is a B cell product (Type I), or cell-mediated by IgG, which is a T or macrophage cell function (Type II). B lymphocytes will also provide IgM and IgG antibodies, which may express themselves in the form of antigen-antibody complexes. These could lead to autoimmune diseases or to cytotoxic reactions. Other considerations of concern relate to the source of the immunocompetent cells and the species and strain of animal. Possibly the best sources of immunocompetent cells would be the peripheral blood, followed by the lymph nodes. However, if the detection system is to be effective a large quantity of cells is needed, particularly because such a small proportion will be stimulated. The selection of the spleen as a source of cells provides easy access to large quantities of cells. The spleen also contains all the necessary cells to mount an immune response. The guinea pig and the mouse were selected because they represent the opposite ends of the continuum with respect to their ability to demonstrate cutaneous reaction to small chemical substances (1, 2). If the differences between the two species are a function of the release of vasoactive substances rather than lymphocyte nonreactivity, then the mouse would be used to provide the immunocompetent cells. This would open up the whole area of genetics involved in the reactivity to cutaneous sensitizing agents, which would eventually provide insight into differences in cutaneous reactivity in humans.

MATERIALS AND METHODS

Experimental Animals

Camm Hartley female guinea pigs were obtained from Camm Laboratories and had a weight range between 200 and 400 g. Balb/c male mice (20-25 g) obtained from Indiana Laboratories were used. All animals were maintained on Purina Laboratory show and tap water *ad libitum* and were housed in environmentally controlled facilities (23 $\pm$0.5°C, 65% R.H.) with controlled 12 hr light-dark cycle.

Spleen Cells

Suspensions of cells were prepared by dicing the spleen on a 100-mesh stainless steel screen and then pressing the material through the screen with the plunger from a 10 cc disposable plastic syringe. The cells were flushed through the screen with RPMI 1640 media and then washed twice in the same media. The splenocytes were resuspended to 2.5×10^7/ml in RPMI 1640 supplemented with a 5% fetal calf serum.

Incubation System

Limbro microtiter plates were employed. Each well contained 200 μl of cells (5×10^6 cells), 10 μl of the sensitizing agents, and 10 μl of the radioisotopic leucine or thymidine. [^{3}H] leucine was used as an index of protein synthesis and [^{3}H] thymidine was used for measuring DNA synthesis. In all experiments the precursors were added 48 hr after initiation of the culture. All culture plates were checked for microbial contamination prior to harvest. The cells were harvested with an Otto Hillar cell harvester which allows for trapping the cells on filter paper, washing them with media, and then precipitating the macromolecules with 10% trichloracetic acid. The acid precipitable material was collected on 5 mm filter paper which was added to a liquid scintillation vial containing 10 ml toluene liquiflor scintillation fluid and counted in a Beckman Scintillation Counter Model LS3133T. Cell numbers were determined electronically on a Counter Model ZB1. Viability was assessed by trypan blue exclusion.

Sensitization Procedures

Dinitrochlorobenzene (DNCB) was employed as the sensitizing agent. Guinea pig sensitization was accomplished by a single 0.1 ml intradermal injection of 0.01% DNCB. Challenge was given 7 days later. Ten injections of DNCB gave no better results than a single injection. The mouse was similarly treated but no skin reaction occurred.

RESULTS

Our first consideration was to determine the length of time mouse lympocytes could be maintained in culture. Mouse spleen cells at 2.5×10^7 cell/ml were placed in microtiter wells and cell number and viability measured out through day 7. Table 1 shows the changes in number and viability as a function of the incubation time. There was no significant change in cell number out through day 4 and cell viability decreased from 99 to 70% over this time period. Cell number increased 1.6-fold on days 5, 6, and 7, and cell viability decreased markedly to 7%. These data, and those obtained from a comparable study on guinea pig lymphocytes, suggest the use of an incubation period of 4 days.

The effect of DNCB (10^{-5} to 10^{-11} M) on the number and

TABLE 1

*Changes in Mouse Spleen Cell Number and Viability as a
Function of Incubation Time*

Time, days	Cells X 10^{6a}	% Change	Viability[b]
0	27.7 ± .8		99
1	25.4 ± 1	− 8	78
2	30.8 ± .9	+11	78
3	22.4 ± 2	−19	72
4	28.0 ± 3	+ 1	70
5	40.0 ± 1	+44	20
6	41.0 ± 5	+48	15
7	47.7 ± 5	+72	7

[a]Mean ± S.E. derived from eight cultures,

[b]Viability determined by trypan blue exclusion.

viability of spleen cells from normal mouse cells is shown
in Table 2. DNCB was added to the microtiter wells at the
same time as the cells. Although variation was observed,
there was no pronounced decrease in the cell number at any
concentration of DNCB. Viability of the lymphocytes as determined by trypan blue exclusion was between 63 and 70%.
We concluded from this experiment that DNCB had no direct
lymphocyte cytotoxicity. Table 3 shows the effect of DNCB
on leucine incorporation into protein. Again there was considerable variation in the experiment but the general trend
between 10^{-5} M and $10^{-11}M$ DNCB was a decrease of leucine incorporation. This is seen in a 76% decrease in incorporation
at 10^{-6} M, 62% at 10^{-8} M and 47% at 10^{-10} M. This decrease
in leucine incorporation was seen in a number of other experiments on unsensitized mouse spleen cells but was not
seen in unsensitized guinea pig cells. A dose-dependent decrease in DNA synthesis as measured by tritiated thymidine
incorporation into DNA was also seen in unsensitized mouse
spleen cells (Table 4). DNCB 10^{-4} M showed cytotoxicity and
must be disregarded in this experiment. DNCB at 10^{-5} M

TABLE 2

Unsensitized Mouse Spleen Cells: Effect of DNCB on Spleen Cell Numbers[a]

DNCB[b]	Cells X 10^6/ml[c]	% Change
Control	9.6 ± 2	
10^{-11}	8.8 ± 1	- 8
10^{-10}	14.6 ± 2	+52
10^{-9}	8.0 ± 8	- 7
10^{-8}	15.0 ± 3	+56
10^{-7}	14.1 ± 3	+47
10^{-6}	$18.3 \pm .9$	+91
10^{-5}	8.8 ± 1	- 8

[a]Spleen cells were incubated with DNCB for 48 hr and cell number determined.

[b]Molar concentration of DNCB.

[c]Mean $\pm$ S.E. derived from eight cultures.

to 10^{-11} M showed inhibition up to 59%. The cell number did not change dramatically except in the cultures receiving 10^{-11} M DNCB. Here there was a 2-fold increase in the number of cells but there was a high variance in the eight cultures.

In contrast to mouse spleen cells, unsensitized guinea pig spleen cells responded to DNCB by showing an increase in [^{3}H]lecuine incorporation into protein (Table 5). Concentrations of DNCB 10^{-5} M to 10^{-11} M gave increases of 18, 17, 47, 35, 27, and 41%, respectively. Cell number remained relatively constant at all concentrations of DNCB. Cell viability in this experiment was between 66 and 80%. In data not shown, the incorporation of [^{3}H]thymidine in the DNA was not as marked as was that of [^{3}H]leucine in unsensitized spleen cells. Only at concentrations of 5×10^{-5} M was there any significant change, but at this concentration most of the cells were killed, as manifested by a low level of viability (Table 6). The differences in reactivity of the guinea pig spleen cells may be a function of the time in

TABLE 3

Unsensitized Mouse Spleen Cells: Effect of DNCB on
[^{3}H]Leucine Incorporation[a]

DNCB[b]	DPM/10^6 Cells[c]	% Change
0	172 $\pm$	
10^{-5}	106 $\pm$ 9	-38
10^{-6}	42 $\pm$ 17	-76
10^{-7}	138 $\pm$ 10	-20
10^{-8}	66 $\pm$ 6	-62
10^{-9}	163 $\pm$ 18	- 5
10^{-10}	92 $\pm$ 8	-47
10^{-11}	96 $\pm$ 11	-44

[a]Spleen cells were incubated with DNCB for 48 hr followed
by a 24 hr pulse of DNCB.

[b]Molar concentration of DNCB.

[c]Mean $\pm$ S.E. derived from eight cultures.

which the pulses occurred. The leucine pulse was given 48
hr after DNCB. This may be too late and a more pronounced
increase may be seen at 24 hr.

The effects of DNCB on spleen cells from DNCB sensitized
guinea pigs are summarized in Table 7. The spleen cells
were incubated with DNCB for 48 hr followed by a 24 hr
[^{3}H]thymidine pulse. Concentrations between 10^{-6} M and
10^{-10} M produced a dose-dependent decrease in thymidine incorporation. Concentrations of 10^{-5} M and 5 x 10^{-5} M caused
an increase in thymidine uptake. However, at 5 x 10^{-5} there
was a cytotoxicity due to the DNCB. Two problems may be inherent in this particular experiment. (1) The timing of the
pulse of thymidine with respect to the challenge of DNCB (at
48 hours) may be past the peak time when DNA synthesis would
be going on. (2) Concentration of DNCB between 10^{-5} M and
5 x 10^{-5} M may be needed to pick up the increase in DNA
synthesis.

TABLE 4

Unsensitized Mouse Spleen Cells: Effect of DNCB on [H]Thymidine Incorporation[a]

DNCB[b]	DPM/10 Cells[c]	% Change	Cells X 10^6/ml[c]	% Change
0	237 ± 17		2.3 ± .6	
10^{-4}	509 ± 55	+115	0.7 ± .02	+30
10^{-5}	130 ± 13	− 45	2.8 ± 1.2	−22
10^{-6}	133 ± 20	− 44	1.9 ± .3	− 7
10^{-7}	248 ± 46	+ 5	1.7 ± .2	−26
10^{-8}	136 ± 3	− 43	2.3 ± .4	− 0
10^{-9}	184 ± 9	− 22	1.9 ± .4	−17
10^{-10}	216 ± 18	− 9	1.5 ± .4	−35
10^{-11}	98 ± 11	−59	4.4 ± 1.1	−91

[a] Spleen cells were incubated with DNCB for 48 hr followed by a 24 hr pulse with [^{3}H] thymidine.

[b] Molar concentration of DNCB.

[c] Mean ± S.E. derived from eight cultures.

TABLE 5

Unsensitized Guinea Pig Spleen Cells: Effect of DNCB on [³H]Leucine Incorporation and Cell Number[a]

DNCB[b]	[³H]Leucine DMP/10⁶ Cells[c]	% Change	Cells X 10⁶/ml[c]	% Change
0	52 ± 9		13.7 ± 1	
5 x 10⁻⁵	42 ± 4	-19	15.9 ± 2	+16
10⁻⁵	66 ± 5	+27	12.6 ± 1	- 8
10⁻⁶	66 ± 6	+23	13.5 ± 1	- 2
10⁻⁷	98 ± 4	+88	10.8 ± 2	-21
10⁻⁸	80 ± 4	+54	12.2 ± 1	-11
10⁻⁹	71 ± 2	+36	13.1 ± 1	- 4
10⁻¹⁰	88 ± 7	+69	10.7 ± 1	-22

[a] Spleen cells were incubated with DNCB for 48 hr followed by a 24 hr pulse with [³H]leucine.

[b] Molar concentration of DNCB.

[c] Mean ± S.E. derived from eight cultures.

TABLE 6

Effect of DNCB on Spleen Cells from DNCB-Sensitized Guinea Pigs[a]

DNCB[b]	DPM/10⁶ Cells[c]	% Change	Cells X 10⁶/ml[c]	% Change
Control	6 ± .8		48 ± 13	
10^{-10}	18 ± 4	+200	39 ± 1	-19
10^{-9}	14 ± 5	+133	41 ± 4	-15
10^{-8}	8 ± 2	+ 33	42 ± 5	-13
10^{-7}	10 ± 3	+ 67	48 ± 3	0
10^{-6}	5 ± 1	- 17	44 ± 1	- 8
10^{-5}	11 ± 5	+ 83	38 ± 8	-21
5×10^{-5}	194 ± 46	+223	2 ± 2	-96

[a] Spleen cells were incubated with DNCB for 48 hr followed by a 24 hr pulse with [³H]leucine.

[b] Molar concentration of DNCB.

[c] Mean ± S.E. derived from eight cultures.

183

TABLE 7

Effect of DNCB on Spleen Cells from DNCB-Sensitized Guinea Pigs[a]

DNCB[b]	DPM/10 Cells[c]	% Change	Cells X 10^6/ml[c]	% Change
Control	59 ± 15		48 ± 13	
10^{-10}	43 ± 5	-27	38 ± 1	-21
10^{-9}	48 ± 12	-19	41 ± 4	-15
10^{-8}	27 ± 4	-54	42 ± 3	-13
10^{-7}	21 ± 5	-64	48 ± 3	0
10^{-6}	19 ± 4	-68	44 ± 1	- 8
10^{-5}	101 ± 44	+71	38 ± 8	-21
5 X 10^{-5}	2924 ± 889	+4856	2 ± 2	-96

[a]Spleen cells were incubated with DNCB for 48 hr followed by a 24 hr [3H]thymidine pulse.

[b]Molar concentration of DNCB.

[c]Mean ± S.E. derived from eight cultures.

The experiments shown in Table 8 were performed in an attempt to determine if the spleen cells from mice which had received intradermal injections of DNCB would respond differently than those of the unsensitized mice. DNCB was administered to mice by the intradermal route 7 days prior to preparation of spleen cells. After 48 hr of incubation with DNCB there was a 24 hr pulse of [^{3}H]leucine. Concentrations of 10^{-9} M and 10^{-8} M DNCB caused a 62% and 56% reduction of leucine incorporation, respectively. DNCB in concentrations of 10^{-9} M, 10^{-8} M, and 5×10^{-5} M caueed 1.8-, 1.7-, and 1.6-fold increases in cell number over the incubation period. There was no significant increase in thymidine incorporation into DNA in this experiment. Again, a major problem in trying to detect greater increases in macromolecular synthesis may be a function of the time when the precursor pulse was given with respect to the challenge of DNCB.

Milner (3) reported that lymph node cells from guinea pigs sensitized by footpad injection with dinitrofluorobenzend (DNFB) responded to *in vitro* stimulation with DNFB-skin protein conjugates. These studies did not include the conjugate nor did they employ serum with clonogenic factors. Better stimulation may result from these additions. This experimental approach may eventually add important information to the conventional patch test for the elicitation of contact dermititis.

We plan to continue to investigate this system in the guinea pig to refine and validate this experimental approach. This will also provide the opportunity to examine cross-reactivity. That is, guinea pigs sensitized to one hapten can be challenged *in vitro* to see if their lymphocytes will respond directly to a second sensitizing agent. The mouse will also be studied so that the genetics of this can be better worked out. We plan to use other sources of lymphocytes, particularly the peripheral blood lymphocytes, for two reasons. The peripheral blood lymphocytes may be more responsive, and we can easily compare the animal data with humans.

SUMMARY

Guinea pig and mouse lymphocytes can be maintained in culture for 4 to 5 days with a 60 to 80% viability and with basal levels of macromolecular synthesis. In naive or unexposed guinea pig lymphocytes, DNCB in concentrations between $10^{-10} M$ and 10^{-5} M gave a slight increase in protein synthesis but not DNA synthesis. This was not the case for mouse lymphocytes. DNCB between 10^{-5} M and 10^{-11} M did not affect cell number of cell viability in naive animals.

TABLE 8

Effect of DNCB on Spleen Cells from DNCB-Treated Mice[a]

DNCB[b]	DPM/10 Cells[c]	% Change	Cells X 10^6/ml[c]	% Change
Control	55 ± 6		11.3 ± 1	
10^{-10}	48 ± 7	-13	12.1 ± .7	+ 7
10^{-9}	21 ± 2	-62	20.0 ± 2	+77
10^{-8}	24 ± 4	-57	18.7 ± 1	+65
10^{-7}	57 ± 5	+ 4	10.4 ± .9	- 8
10^{-6}	54 ± 5	- 2	9.1 ± .4	-20
10^{-5}	30 ± 7	-46	11.3 ± 2	0
5 x 10^{-5}	43 ± 3	-22	18.0 ± 2	+59

[a]Spleen cells were incubated with DNCB for 48 hr followed by a 24 hr pulse with [^{3}H]leucine.

[b]Molar concentration of DNCB.

[c]Mean ± S.E. derived from eight cultures.

There was no increase in lymphocyte cell number from sensitized guinea pig lymphocyte cultures when challenged *in vitro* with DNCB. In fact, there was a decrease consistent with *in vivo* findings. This system offers the opportunity to separate the immunocompetent cells and to ask them to respond to a potential cutaneous sensitizing agent.

REFERENCES

1. Crowle, A. J. (1975). Delayed hypersensitivity in the mouse. *Adv. Immunol.* *20*:197.
2. Mills, J. A. (1966). The immunologic significance of antigen induced lymphocyte transformation *in vitro*. *J. Immunol.* 97:239.
3. Milner, J. E. (1970). *In vitro* lymphocyte responses in contact hypersensitivity. *J. Invest. Dermatol.* *55*:34.

The Value and Significance
of Carcinogenic, Mutagenic, and Teratogenic Tests

David J. Brusick

Department of Genetics
Litton Bionetics, Inc.
Kensington, Maryland

Testing for the carcinogenic, mutagenic, and teratogenic (CM&T) effects of chemicals is difficult in itself, but the task is considerably more difficult for topically applied materials. In fact, with the exception of skin-painting procedures utilized in carcinogenicity screening, few reports are available describing attempts to determine CM&T effects by dermal application. Parameters such as the absorption and the bioavailability of the compound to the target sites involved in these three phenomena necessitate the development of new and relevant model systems. For example, the area of topical application may be a target site for certain lesions such as somatic mutation and carcinogenesis, whereas absorption and systemic distribution of the substance or an active metabolite will be necessary for the induction of germinal cell mutations. In addition to absorption and systemic distribution, the production of terata (abnormal offspring) requires the transport of the substance across the placenta. Another important factor in CM&T testing is the level of exposure. While definite toxic and sensitivity thresholds can be measured with reasonable accuracy in animal models or human clinical tests, the same is not true for CM&T events. Positive effects for these three end points can be obtained at exposure levels well below concentrations required to demonstrate the overt toxic or skin irritation effects that normally alert investigators to the presence of potentially harmful effects. Therefore, to determine the potential CM&T effects of cutaneously applied substances, sensitive test procedures which take into account not only the problems of exposure, absorption, and bioavailability but also the close relationship among mechanisms involved in producing CM&T effects must be developed.

CORRELATION OF CARCINOGENIC, MUTAGENIC, AND TERATOGENIC RESPONSE TO CHEMICALS

During the past few years the possibility of establishing a direct link between the processes of mutagenesis and carcinogenesis has been enhanced by the results of comparative investigations with chemicals exhibiting both properties (3, 7, 14, 17, 18, 19, 23, 24, 25) and by investigations into the molecular mechanisms involved in malignant transformation of cultured mammalian cells (4, 7, 8, 24).

It has been established for a wide range of chemical classes that most animal carcinogens are also mutagens or produce mutagenic metabolites (18, 19). The data base from which this correlation has been developed consists of several hundred chemicals which include agents known to induce cancer in test animals and humans and chemicals considered to be noncarcinogenic. The results of the studies indicate a positive correlation of approximately 0.90 between carcinogenicity and mutagenicity (18) and a positive correlation of approximately 0.98 between noncarcinogenicity and nonmutagenicity (1, 18, 20), where agreement can be reached on the carcinogenicity or noncarcinogenicity of a compound. To be certain, the designations noncarcinogen and nonmutagen cannot be considered unequivocal but are made in the context of available testing techniques. There is in this mutagen:carcinogen correlation a definite gray area of apparent inconsistency, especially among chemicals whose structural configurations are very similar to those of established animal carcinogens. There are several possible explanations for the lack of complete correlation between the mutagenic and carcinogenic properties of such chemicals, some of which are listed below:

1. Specific differences in intracellular biochemistry between prokaryotic bacterial cells and eukaryotic animal cells may permit certain types of chemicals to exhibit mutagenic activity in microbial DNA with no similar response to mammalian cells.
2. Chemicals with weak carcinogenic potential may not be detected in bioassay procedures without tremendously increasing the sample size of treated individuals. How-

ever, the same compound may exhibit mutagenic activity in microbial assays with *Salmonella*, for example.

3. It is not uncommon for samples of noncarcinogenic analogs or isomers of established carcinogens to contain small concentrations of the carcinogenic substance. In some situations, this contamination is sufficient to produce a mutagenic response in microbial assays (B.N. Ames, personal communication).

4. Data from some carcinogenicity bioassay studies may have been erroneous or insufficient to produce an accurate assessment of the actual potential of the compound, thus affecting the reliability of the correlation.

5. There are certain classes of chemicals which promote the initiation of cancer in animals but which are not themselves initiators. Data from microbial short-term mutagenesis tests indicate that such "indirect carcinogens" will not be mutagenic.

There are certainly other reasons preventing a complete match between mutagenesis and carcinogenesis; however, the correlation as it presently stands strongly suggests a more than coincidental relationship between the two phenomena (19, 25, 27, 28).

For certain chemicals the carcinogenic and mutagenic correlation can be extended into a carcinogenic, mutagenic, and teratogenic (CM&T) correlation (Table 1). The reason for this seems to be that there is a genetic component to the production of terata (13, 21, 29, 30). However, a correlation for CM&T similar to the relationship between carcinogenicity and mutagenicity cannot be expected because of the diversity of mechanisms leading to a teratogenic end point (30). Many of these teratogenic mechanisms such as enzyme inhibition, membrane alterations, metabolic imbalances, and endocrine dysfunctions are not under direct genetic regulation; therefore, it could be extremely misleading to attempt to use short-term mutagenicity assays for the presumptive identification of teratogens without confirmation using appropriate animal models. About the most one can determine is that there appears to be a genetic element in teratogenicity and that mutagens might be suspect teratogens. From a theoretical point of view, those agents capable of producing small deletions, point mutations, or mitotic recombination might be the most typical teratogenic mutagens because these may well result in cell division problems, nondisjunction, homozygosity, and ploidy changes. Many chromosomal alterations of a large proportion result in dominant lethality and not teratogenicity. However, the relationship between mutagenic and teratogenic effects has not been either qualitatively or quantitatively defined and many classes of genetic effects might be involved.

TABLE 1

A Comparison of the Carcinogenic, Mutagenic, and Teratogenic Effects of Several Chemical Classes[a]

Agent	Mutagen	Carcinogen	Teratogen
Nitrogen mustard	+	+	+
Cyclophosphamide	+	+	+
Triethylenemelamine (TEM)	+	+	+
6-Mercaptopurine	+	+	+
Hycanthone	+	+	+
Captan	+	+	+
Folpet	+	+	+
X-irradiation	+	+	+
Cigarette smoke (condensate products)	+	+	(+)
Triazenes	+	+	+
Androgenic hormones	−	?	+
Rubella virus	−	−	+
Quinacrine	(+)	−	+
Halothane	(+)	?	(+)
5-Fluorouracil	−	−	+
Cytosine arabinoside	(+)	−	+
Hydroxyurea	−	−	+
Methotrexate	(+)	(+)	+
Actinomycin D	−	−	+

TABLE 1 - Cont'd.

A Comparison of the Carcinogenic, Mutagenic, and Teratogenic Effects of Several Chemical Classes[a]

Agent	Mutagen	Carcinogen	Teratogen
Benzene	-	-	+
Urethane	-	+	+
Colchicine	-	-	+
Chlorpromazine	(+)	-	+

[a]Among a diverse group of recognized teratogens it can be seen that the relationship between CM&T holds only about 50% of the compounds. The remaining agents that are teratogenic appear to act through nongenetic mechanisms or possibly multiple mechanisms some of which may have an indirect genetic basis.

( ) = data questionable, conflicting, or results obtained only under very specialized treatment procedures.

PROBLEMS ASSOCIATED WITH EVALUATING TOPICAL AGENTS FOR CARCINOGENIC, MUTAGENIC, AND TERATOGENIC EFFECTS

The carcinogenic, mutagenic, and teratogenic response obtained in animals is a combination of a chemical's toxic potential combined with its opportunity to impact on the target site. For studies of cutaneously applied substances these factors become even more important, especially when considering germ cell mutations or teratogenicity. Except for the animal skin-painting experiments to determine carcinogenic potential, very little work has gone into the development of model systems to measure carcinogenic, mutagenic, and teratogenic effects of cutaneously applied substances.

Negative results following dermal application of chemicals may be due to the absence of a toxic effect or to the fact that a potentially toxic compound did not reach the target organ. Thus, a compound might be judged toxic following intramuscular injection but may be safe when applied to the skin. Access of topically applied substances to various target sites is dependent on their ability to pass certain

protective barriers, namely: (a) dermal absorption;
(b) systemic distribution, metabolism, detoxification; and
(c) placental/gonadal penetration.

Absorption of Cutaneously Applied Substances

Dermal penetration of topically applied materials is of
course necessary before a critical factor of the test material can be detected or measured in blood. Species differences in the level and rate of topical absorption of various
chemicals are well known and increase the complexity of using
this route of administration and extrapolation of the results to man, For example, data shown in Table 2 illustrate
the spectra of responses from several mammalian species for
hydrocarbon carcinogenesis using cutaneous and subcutaneous
administrations (29). The skin is also a metabolic organ a
and thus the biotransformation of the applied substance to
metabolic derivatives must be considered.

Systemic Disposition of Cutaneously Applied Substances

Absorption of the material or its metabolites into the
systemic blood circulation allows potential exposure of many
organs to the substances. However, after absorption the
material is placed in environments where additional metabolism can occur, resulting in activation or detoxification
(5). These factors, plus concentration and excretion by the
kidney, permit the actual systemic exposure period for a
given chemical to vary tremendously. Nevertheless, under
certain conditions somatic mutation and neoplasia may possibly result from cutaneous application.

Placental/Gonadal Penetration of Cutaneously Applied Substances

Two critical end points (mutation and terata) may be affected by exposure of the gonadal and intrauterine environments to carcinogens, mutagens, and teratogens. It is interesting from an evolutionary standpoint that systems involved in maintaining the hereditary integrity of a species
are equipped with extra-protective systems isolating them
from systemic exposure inflicted on other organs. In the
gonads, and especially the testes, there is a blood-testicu-
lar barrier which restricts penetration of specific chemicals
into the gonadal environment (10, 30). The placenta acts as
a selective barrier to a number of compounds although it is
known that many chemicals, viruses, and immune components
pass through from the maternal environment to the intrauterine environment by simple diffusion, active transport,

TABLE 2

*Comparison of Species Differences in the Carcinogenesis
Response to Polycyclic Aromatic Hydrocarbons Administered
Cutaneously*[a]

Species	Testing system	
	By skin painting	By subcutaneous injection
Mouse	+ + + + +	+ + + + +
Rabbit	+ + + +	+
Rat	+ +	+ + + + + +
Guinea pig	+ +	+ +
Hamster	+ + +	+ + +
Fowl	+	+ + + +
Dog	+ +	?+
Man	+ + +	?+

[a]From I. Berenblum, *Carcinogenesis as a Biological
Problem,* North-Holland/American Elsevier, Amsterdam, 1974,
with permission of the publisher.

penocytosis, and leakage (30). It is also known that the
placenta possesses metabolic capabilities (5, 6, 8, 15, 30).
    Therefore when considering that an effect is the product
of toxic potential and opportunity to reach the target organ, assaying for CM&T effects produced by cutaneously
applied substances must incorporate a great number of assumptions and difficult measurements to determine the actual
target organ dose. Simple measurements of blood levels may
suffice for the determination of exposure of some potential
targets but certainly not for gonadal mutagenesis, teratogenesis, or intrauterine mutagenesis. The need to develop good
model systems is obvious.

SOME CURRENT PROBLEMS IN CUTANEOUS EXPOSURE RELATED TO
CARCINOGENIC, MUTAGENIC, AND TERATOGENIC EFFECTS

During the past 3 years several situations have arisen
regarding the potential safety of certain substances which
come in contact with the skin of man. In 1975 Ames (2) reported that most commercial oxidative hair dyes were mutagenic in tests using microbial indicator organisms. This
observation was followed by similar conclusions regarding
the hair dyes sold in Great Britain and Japan (1, 26). It
has also been noted that some of the dye products are absorbed through human skin (16), and mutagenic products can
be identified in the urine of mice and rats following dye
application (Brusick, unpublished). As a result, the question of the potential carcinogenic, mutagenic, and teratogenic (CM&T) effects in exposed individuals has received
substantial publicity.

More recently certain flame-retardant compounds used to
impregnate children's clothing and other items have been
reported, on the basis of microbial assays, to be mutagenic
(1, 20, Brusick, unpublished). Again the questions of possible dermal absorption and systemic distribution of these
substances have been raised with respect to CM&T effects.
Little is known regarding cutaneous absorption and systemic
disposition of these substances, and they remain as potential problems.

Finally, there has been substantial activity in the development of topical antimicrobials and especially topical
antiviral substances in recent years. The antiviral compounds are of most interest in that they generally consist
of compounds which interfere with normal nucleic acid metabolism. This class of compounds could certainly be expected
to have potential CM&T activity and will require adequate
evaluation before they are used in a large-scale basis.

The potential for inflicting CM&T effects in mammals has
been either demonstrated or strongly inferred for each of
these three types of materials and each represents an area
of cutaneous chemical application, encompassing hundreds or
thousands of untested substances, for which good model test
systems to assess safety are not available.

DEVELOPMENT OF A MODEL ASSAY SYSTEM

The application of certain short-term *in vitro* or *in
vivo* tests for predicting CM&T effects could play a significant role in the construction of a relevant toxicological
profile on a given substance. Materials tested for mutagenicity in the Ames *Salmonella*/microsome assay or an *in*

vitro cell transformation assay can identify specific potential, but extension of the identified potential into the
likelihood of a mutagenic or carcinogenic effect being induced *in vivo* by the material requires a greater insight into
the biodynamics of the agents. Figure 1 is a composite of
several short-term *in vivo* and *in vitro* assays coupled with
certain pharmacological test procedures. This battery of
assays should be potentially useful in determining the possibility that a compound may induce molecular alterations in
critical target molecules as well as provide insight into the

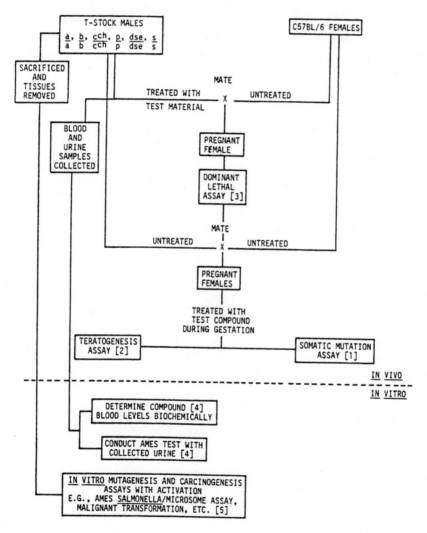

*Fig. 1. Proposed composite test system to screen for CM&T
potential in chemicals.*

ability of the substance to impact on the gonadal and intrauterine environments.

The critical feature of this composite series of tests
is the use of a T-strain of mice homozygous for several coat
color genes (non-agonti, *aa*; pink-eye, *pp*; brown, *bb*;
dilute, *dd*; chinchilla, $c^{ch}c^{ch}$; spotted, *ss*; short-ear, *sese*)
(6, 22). Employing this mouse strain in specific assays
permits the following series of end points to be detected
and quantitied:

1. Intrauterine somatic mutations may be induced in developing embryos. During intrauterine development, mouse embryos resulting from a T shock X C57BL/6 (wild-type for
   all the alleles) cross are exposed to a test chemical for
   5 days during the fifth to the tenth day of pregnancy.
   Mutation at any of the coat color alleles derived from
   the C57BL/6 stock to a recessive allele in a pigment cell
   produces a patch of coat color different from the anticipated black color (6). This can be detected by examination of a relatively small number (less than 200) of offspring. The number of chemicals which have been examined
   in this type of assay is approximately ten and includes
   both frameshift and base substitution mutagens (6, 11,
   22). This type of mutation assay is extremely valuable
   in measuring the ability of a chemical to cross the
   barriers described previously.
2. Simultaneously with the performance of the previous test,
   a subgroup of the treated pregnant females could be
   examined for the presence of terata. These two assays,
   if run jointly, could provide valuable toxicology data
   on the chemical, in addition to measuring the correlation between the induction of somatic mutation and tera-
   togenity.
3. A modification of the above procedures, in which T-strain
   males are treated for 5 days and then mated weekly to
   virgin females in a dominant lethal protocol, could be
   used to assess potential germ cell risk to chromosomal
   effects induced by the test substance.
4. Blood and urine can be collected over several days following acute exposure or during the period of subchronic
   exposure to the test chemical and can then be examined
   for: (a) blood levels of the test chemical and (b) the
   presence of a mutagenic substance or its metabolites in
   the urine by application of the Ames assay (9). These
   two sensitive assays can be used to investigate bioavailability of the agents as well as excretion and
   conjugation.
5. The tests described above can be supplemented with *in
   vitro* assays including the Ames *Salmonella*/microsome

assay and malignant transformation of cultured rodent
cells (24) to generate a balanced set of molecular
toxicological data.

This array of data could be used in the overall toxicological evaluation of the test substance to predict not only
the potential of CM&T effects but also the probability of
these events occurring in exposed mammals. The composite
test series is quite amenable to screening cutaneously
applied substances. The overall cost of performing such a
composite series of tests would be approximately $20,000 per
compound and require a testing time of only 3 to 4 months.
   It can be concluded that the proposed model is a feasible
(all the proposed tests are currently being conducted) and
powerful test battery with which important questions concerning the carcinogenic, mutagenic, and teratogenic potential of a compound can be economically answered in a relevant manner using sound scientific procedures.

REFERENCES

1. Ames, B. N. Personal communication.
2. Ames, B. N., Kammen, H. O., and Yamasaki, E. (1975).
   Hair dyes are mutagenic: Identification of a variety of
   mutagenic ingredients. *Proc. Nat. Acad. Sci. U.S.A. 72:*
   2423.
3. Ames, B. N., McCann, J., and Yamasaki, E. (1975).
   Methods for detecting carcinogens and mutagens with the
   Salmonella/mallalian-microsome mutagenicity test.
   *Mutat. Res. 31:*347.
4. Berenblum, I. (1974). *Carcinogenesis as a Biological
   Problem.* Amsterdam, North-Holland.
5. Conney, A. H., and Burns, J. J. (1972). Metabolic interactions among environmental chemicals and drugs.
   *Science 178:*576.
6. Davidson, G. E., and Dawson, G. W. P. (1976). Chemically-
   induced presumed somatic mutations in the mouse. *Mutat.
   Res. 38:*115.
7. DiPaolo, J. A., Nelson, R. L., and Donovan, P. J. (1972).
   In vitro transformation of Syrian hamster embryo cells
   by diverse chemical carcinogens. *Nature*(London), *New
   Biol. 235:*287.
8. DiPaolo, J. A., Nelson, R. L., Donovan, P. H., and
   Evans, C. H. (1973). Host-mediated *in vivo-in vitro*
   assay for chemical carcinogenesis. *Arch. Pathol. 95:*
   380.
9. Durston, W. E., and Ames, B. N. (1974). A simple method
   for the detection of mutagens in urine: Studies with

the carcinogen 2-acetylaminofluorene. *Proc. Nat. Acad. Sci. U.S.A.* *71*:737.

10. Ehling, U. H. (1971). Comparison of radiation and chemically-induced lethal mutations in male mice. *Mutat. Res.* *11*:35.

11. Fahrig, R. (1975). The mammalian spot test, a sensitive *in vivo* method for the detection of genetic alterations in somatic cells of mice. Abst. Ka-7, European Environmental Mutagen Society Meeting, Oct. 19-22, Florence, Italy.

12. Flynn, E. J., Lynch, M., and Zannoni, V. G. (1972). Species differences and drug metabolism. *Biochem. Pharmacol.* *21*:2577.

13. Fraser, F. C. (1969). Gene-environment interactions in the production of cleft palate. In *Method for Teratological Studies in Experimental Animals and Man,* eds. H. Nishimura and J.R. Miller, p. 34-39. Tokyo, Igalsu Shoin.

14. Isono, K., and Yourno, J. (1974). Chemical carcinogens as frameshift mutagens: *Salmonella* DNA sequence sensitive to mutagenesis by polycyclic carcinogens. *Proc. Nat. Acad. Sci. U.S.A.* *71*:1612.

15. Juchau, M. R. (1972). Mechanisms of drug biotransformation reactions in placenta. *Fed. Proc. Fed. Am. Soc. Exp. Biol.* *31*:48.

16. Kiese, M., and Rauscher, E. (1968). The absorption of P-toluenediamine through human skin in hair dyeing. *Toxicol. Appl. Pharmacol.* *13*:325.

17. McCalla, D. R., and Voutsinos, D. (1974). On the mutagenicity of nitrofurans. *Mutat. Res.* *26*:3.

18. McCann, J., Choi, E., Yamasaki, E., and Ames, B. N. (1975). Detection of carcinogens as mutagens in the *Salmonella*/microsome test: Assay of 300 chemicals. *Proc. Nat. Acad. Sci. U.S.A.* *72*:5135.

19. Miller, E. C., and Miller, J. A. (1971). The mutagenicity of chemical carcinogens: Correlation, problems and interpretations. In *Chemical Mutagens: Principles and Methods for Their Detection*, ed. A. Hollaender, p. 83. New York and London, Plenum Press.

20. Rosenkranz, H. Personal communication.

21. Roux, C., Emerit, I., and Taillemite, J. (1971). Chromosome breakage and teratogenesis. *Teratology, 4*: 303.

22. Russel, L. B. (1976). The *in vivo* coat-color somatic-mutation method in chemical mutagenesis studies in the mouse. Abst. Cb-10, Seventh Annual Meeting, Environment Mutagen Society, March 12-15, Atlanta, Georgia.

23. Slater, E. E., Anderson, M. D., and Rosenkranz, H. S. (1971). Rapid detection of mutagens and carcinogens.

Cancer Res. *31:*970.

24. Stolz, D. R., Poirier, L. A., Irving, C. C., Stich, H. E., Weisburger, J. H., and Grice, H. C. (1974). Evaluation of short-term tests for carcinogenicity. *Toxicol. Appl. Pharmacol.* *29:*157.

25. Teranishi, K., Hamada, K., and Watanabe, H. (1975). Quantitative relationship between carcinogenicity and mutagenicity of polyaromatic hydrocarbons in *Salmonella typhimurium* mutants. *Mutat. Res.* *31:*97.

26. Venitt, S. (1975). Mutagenic effects of hair colourants on bacteria and mammalian cells. Abst. Ea-5, European Environmental Mutagen Society Meeting, Oct. 19-22, Florence, Italy.

27. Weekes, U. Y. (1975). Metabolism of dimethylnitrosamine to mutagenic intermediates by kidney microsomal enzymes and correlation with reported host susceptibility to kidney tumors. *J. Nat. Cancer Inst.* *55:*1199.

28. Weekes, U., and Brusick, D. J. (1975). *In vitro* activation of chemical mutagens. II. The relationships among mutagen formation, metabolism and carcinogenicity for dimethyl- and diethylnitrosamine in the liver, kidneys and lungs of BALB/cJ, C57Bl/6J and RF/J mice. *Mutat. Res.* *31:*175.

29. Wernick, T., Lanman, B. M., and Iraux, J. L. (1976). Chronic toxicity, teratologic and reproduction studies with hair dyes. *Toxicol. Appl. Pharmacol.* (in press).

30. Wilson, J. B. (1973). *Environment and Birth Defects.* New York, Academic Press.

The Chemistry and Toxicology of Hair Dyes

Clyde M. Burnett and John F. Corbett

Clairol Research Laboratory
Stamford, Connecticut

The use of synthetic dyes for coloring human hair dates from 1883, when Monnet (1) patented a process for coloring hair by application of a freshly prepared mixture of a solution of p-phenylenediamine and hydrogen peroxide. This process, forming the basis of the so-called permanent hair colorant, is extensively used today.

In the last 12 months, hair dyes have been the subject of considerable publicity as a result of a finding that some of the ingredients are mutagenic towards a special strain of *Salmonella typhimurium*, giving rise to the claim that they might be carcinogenic. In view of this, it seemed timely to review the chemistry and toxicology of hair dyes.

Modern hair coloring systems can conveniently be divided into three categories: temporary, semipermanent, and permanent (2). These three categories are characterized by the type of dye employed, the method of application, and the permanence of the resulting color.

TEMPORARY HAIR COLORANTS

Temporary hair colorants, often referred to as "color rinses," make use of acid dyes of the type used in wool dyeing. These are fairly high molecular weight species which deposit on the surface of the hair fiber, rather than penetrate into the cortex.

Few, if any, of the commercial products rely on a single dye. Rather, the shade is achieved by using a mixture of dyes (Figure 1). These dyes, in an aqueous solution containing a small amount of surfactant, are applied to the roots of the hair and combed through to the tip. The hair is then set and dried; no rinsing is required.

This type of product is used for adding light colors to gray hair, "toning" gray or bleached hair, or as dramatic "party" colors. Although fast to water, the color can be removed by shampooing.

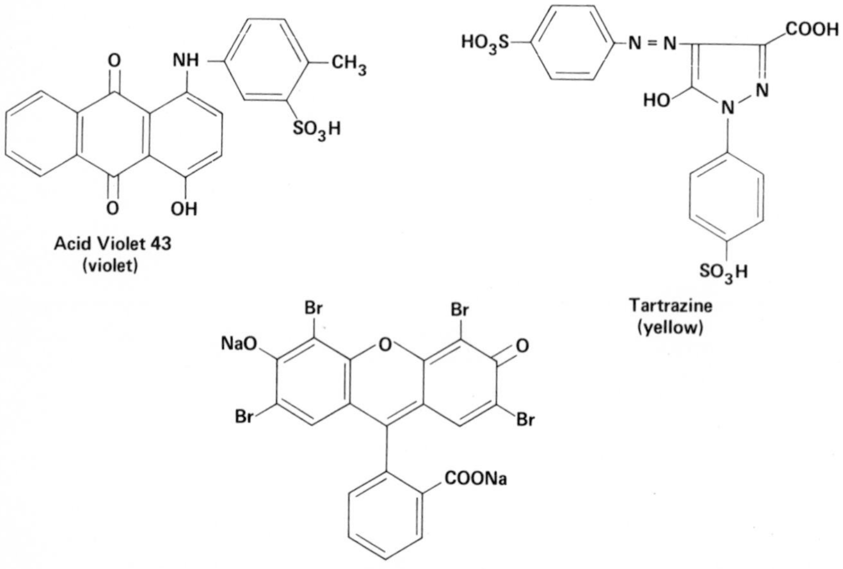
O
NH
CH3
SO3H
O
OH
Acid Violet 43
(violet)
HO3S
N = N
COOH
N
HO
N
SO3H
Tartrazine
(yellow)
Br
Br
NaO
O
O
Br
Br
COONa
Eosin YS
(red)

Fig. 1. Examples of dyes used in temporary hair colorants.

SEMIPERMANENT HAIR COLORANTS

The term "semipermanent" was coined to define hair color products which give a coloration that lasts through five to six shampoos, and do not involve the use of hydrogen peroxide in the color development. This level of wash fastness is achieved by using low molecular weight dyes which are capable of penetrating into the cortex.

Again, natural hair colors cannot be achieved by the use of a single dye species, and it is necessary to blend a number of dyes to attain the desired shade. For example, the color produced by a particular commercial product may result from the presence of nine individual dyes, e.g., four yellows, two reds, one purple, and two violet-blues. This blend is necessary to achieve the desired color and to obtain a match between the color on the root area and that on the more weathered and worn, and thus more permeable, ends.

The dyes used in semipermanent products are mainly nitrophenylenediamines, nitroaminophenols, aminoanthraquinones and, less frequently, azobenzenes. Typical dyes and their colors are shown in Table 1. The dyes are usually dispersed in a shampoo base which is applied to freshly shampooed hair and left on for 20 to 40 minutes before being rinsed out.

TABLE 1

Examples of Dyes Suitable for Use in Semipermanent Hair Colorants

Dye	Chemical Class
2-Nitro-p-phenylenediamine (red)	Nitro
4-Nitro-o-phenylenediamine (yellow)	Nitro
2-Amino-4-nitrophenol (yellow)	Nitro
Picramic acid (orange)	Nitro
N', N^4, N^4-tris(2-hydroxyethyl) 2-nitro-p-phenylenediamine (blue-violet)	Nitro
Disperse blue	Anthraquinone
Disperse red 17	Azo
Disperse violet 4	Anthraquinone
Disperse yellow 1	Nitro

PERMANENT HAIR COLORANTS

Permanent hair colorants are the most important class of

products, accounting for about three out of every four
dollars spent on hair coloring in the United States. In
this system the colored material is produced inside the hair
fiber by oxidation of colorless "intermediates." Since the
hydrogen peroxide used to develop the color is also effective
in bleaching melanin, these systems are unique in their ability to produce lighter shades than the original color of
the hair.

To accomplish the color-forming reactions, three classes
of chemical reactants are required: the primary intermediates, the couplers, and the oxidant. The primary intermediates are the so-called "para" dyes, particularly para-phenylenediamine, para-toluylenediamine, and para-aminophenol.
These materials are capable of undergoing oxidation by the
oxidant, normally hydrogen peroxide, to give benzoquinone
imines. The imines react rapidly with the couplers and/or
an unoxidized "para" to produce indo dyes. The most frequently used couplers are 2,4-diaminoanisole (blue-forming
coupler), resorcinol (green/brown-forming coupler), meta-
aminophenol (magenta/brown color former), and 1-naphthol
(purple blue color former). A more complete list of
intermediates is given in Table 2.

The dye base for oxidation colors is normally built
around an ammonium oleate soap with only a small amount of
detergent. Free ammonia is present to promote the oxidation reaction and the pH of the mixture on the head is about
9.5.

During the past ten years considerable effort has been
devoted to elucidating the mechanism of the color-forming
reactions and the nature of the colored products (3). It has
been shown that the initial reaction involves oxidation of
the primary intermediate, either by hydrogen peroxide or by
oxygen formed by decomposition of hydrogen peroxide inside
the hair fiber, to give a benzoquinone di-imine. The latter
reacts rapidly with one of the couplers to give an indo dye.
Some of these indo dyes are the final colored product in the
hair, while others undergo further reaction to form polymeric
indo compounds.

Some of the more important color-forming reactions are
shown in Figure 2. The chemistry involved can be summarized
as shown in Figure 3.

The oxidation dyes produce fast colors which are not removed by shampooing. In fact, subsequent dyeing is necessitated more by the need to color the new hair growth than by
the fading of the already colored hair. Nevertheless some
off-shade fading, manifest by the development of a red tinge,
is observed, due to slow chemical changes in the indo dyes
(3).

TABLE 2

Colors Produced by Various Components in Permanent Hair Colorants

Colors produced by primary intermediates

Compound	Color on hair
p-Phenylenediamine	Dark brown
p-Toluylenediamine	Light reddish brown
p-Aminodiphenylamine	Dark gray-black
p-Aminophenol	Light auburn
2-Amino-5-hydroxytoluene	Golden blond
5-Amino-2-hydroxytoluene	Reddish blond
o-Aminophenol	Deep gold

Colors produced by p-phenylenediamine in the presence of various couplers

Coupler	Color on hair
None	Dark brown
m-Phenylenediamine	Bluish purple
2,4-Diaminoanisole	Purple-blue
m-Aminophenol	Light brown
4-Methyl-3-aminophenol	Light brown
m-Methoxyphenol	Magenta
6-Methyl-3-aminophenol	Magenta
2,5-Xylenol	Bluish purple
Resorcinol	Greenish brown
Hydroquinone	Light gray-brown
Catechol	Gray-brown

Colors produced by p-aminophenol with various couplers

Coupler	Color on hair
None	Light auburn
m-Phenylenediamine	Blue (at pH 8-11)
m-Aminophenol	Red-brown
6-Methyl-3-aminophenol	Bright orange

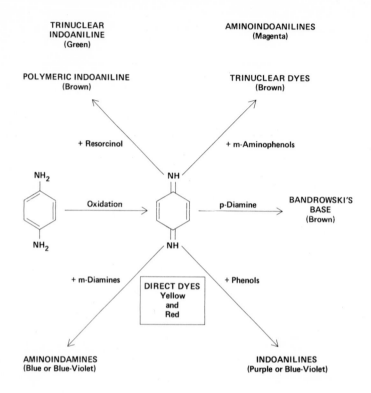

Fig. 2. *Color-forming reactions in oxidative color development.*

DERMATOLOGICAL STUDIES

Para-phenylenediamine, the major component of oxidation hair dyes, is well known to be a sensitizer and to be capable of producing contact dermatitis. In a recent study of sufferers from various dermatoses, 8% showed a reaction when patch tested with p-phenylenediamine (4, 5).

Because of this property, hair colorants carry in the United States, as a legal requirement, instructions for a 24-hr patch test with the intermediates and hydrogen peroxide mixed in the same manner as in use. It indeed seems likely that more sensitization tests have been performed with oxidation colors than with any other material.

It is significant that, while p-phenylenediamine is high on the list of allergens, the incidence of allergic sensitization by oxidation hair dyes is an infrequent and usually mild occurrence.

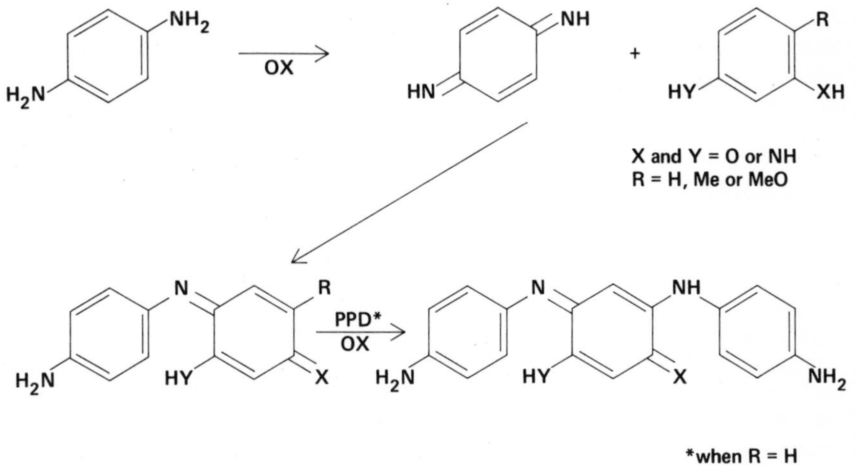

Fig. 3. *The chemistry of oxidative coupling reactions.*

An important difference should be pointed out between patch testing with *p*-phenylenediamine alone and reaction to hair dyes under normal use conditions. In the latter case, contact time is restricted to 30 min with a solution containing less than 3% of *p*-phenylenediamine, and in the presence of an oxidizing agent and couplers, such as resorcinol, 2,4-diaminoanisole, *m*-aminophenol, and *l*-naphthol, which rapidly react with the oxidation products. In fact, under use conditions, the half-life of the di-imine formed by oxidation of the *p*-phenylenediamine is just a few milliseconds, and its concentration never reaches a detectable level (6). Furthermore, little if any Bandrowski's base is formed. It is evident, we believe, that the sensitizing potential, or any other toxicological characteristic of oxidation hair colors, can be meaningfully assessed only by using the total composition, including the hydrogen peroxide, as the test material, rather than using *p*-phenylenediamine or its oxidation products.

In 1973, a booklet published by the Committee of Cutaneous Health and Cosmetics of the AMA gave an estimate that allergic dermatitis due to *p*-phenylenediamine in hair dyes would be one reaction in every 100,000 applications (7). Hair colorants are not a major cause of dermatitis, as judged by the level of incidence reported by dermatologists (although contrary opinions are sometimes expressed) (8).

Industry figures indicate about one allergy complaint for every million units sold. This is probably better than the record for many edible fruits or dairy products!

The end products of the reaction appear to be quite unreactive, a point which is demonstrated by a recent experiment (5) in which 20 people with strong positive patch-test reactions to *p*-phenylenediamine were challenged with hair that had been dyed 24 hr previously with a *p*-phenylenediamine-containing system. None of the 20 showed any reaction to the dyed hair. It was also noted that one of the subjects habitually wore a toupee that had been dyed with *p*-phenylenediamine, while three others wore similarly dyed fur coats.

Finally, practical testimony to the safety record of modern *p*-phenylenediamine hair colors is provided by current European developments. In 1906, the wealth of adverse reactions to hair dyes prompted the German and French governments to place restrictions on the use of *p*-phenylenediamine in hair dyes. Today, under the proposed European Economic Community regulations, concentrations up to 6% of *p*-phenylenediamine will be permitted.

The improved dermatological safety of modern oxidation colors may be ascribed to five factors: (a) present-day raw material manufacturing processes produce *p*-phenylenediamine of very high purity; (b) the availability of stabilized hydrogen peroxide results in proper product performance during application; (c) the proper formulation of the product results in rapid consumption of the intermediate imines which have been suggested as being responsible for the sensitizing property of *p*-phenylenediamine; (d) formulation of the products in a shampoo base ensures more efficient removal of the unused materials at the end of the process; and (e) sale of complete kits ensures use of the proper proportions of reactants.

SYSTEMIC TOXICOLOGY

Although the dermatological properties of hair dye ingredients have been studied for more than 50 years, it is only recently that the systemic toxicity has been considered beyond the level of LD_{50} determination. Interest in systemic toxicity stemmed from the realization that small amounts of some hair dye ingredients can penetrate the skin. Thus Kiese and Rauscher (9) found that about 0.2% of the applied dose of *p*-toluylenediamine was percutaneously absorbed during hair dyeing. This corresponds to a systemic exposure of about 0.1 mg/kg. It has also been reported (10, 10a) that some semipermanent dyes penetrate the skin at low levels and that, in very rare cases, this penetration is sufficient to discolor the urine (11). It is apparent from all these studies that urinary excretion of the absorbed dyes or their metabolites does occur.

In the light of this knowledge, individual companies and the Cosmetic Toiletry and Fragrance Association (CTFA) in the United States have been pursuing a comprehensive testing program for a number of years.

In March 1975, a full-page article appeared in the *New York Times* (12) alleging that the use of hair dyes might cause cancer and/or birth defects. This allegation was based on the work of Ames *et al.*, which was published some months later (13). Ames' group had been developing bacterial screening tests for carcinogens and were using *Salmonella typhimurium* TA 1538. This is a mutant strain which is incapable of synthesizing histidine, is defective in DNA-repair, and has a defective lipopolysaccharide cell wall, rendering it more permeable to test materials. In the test, bacterial colonies will develop if the test chemical causes a frameshift mutation. Ames claims (14) that 90% of the known carcinogens tested give a positive response in this screening test while only a few of the noncarcinogens tested are positive. However, it is important to note that while he found nine oxidation hair dye ingredients to give a positive test (13), these were all aromatic amines and, in addition, three of them also contained nitro groups. Examination of Ames' correlative data (14), in which he used the broadest possible definition of "carcinogen," shows that he obtained 4/12 (i.e., 33%) false positives with aromatic amines, and 3/4 (i.e., 75%) false positives with nitro compounds. In a more recent paper Ames (15) acknowledges that it might be that *S. Typhimurium* contains reductases which are not present in liver or in the *E. coli* of the human gut and that this might give rise to false positives.

Similar bacterial screening tests with hair dyes were reported by Searle *et al.* (16) in England, McPhee (17) in Australia, and Nishioka (18) in Japan. The latter (18) used *E. coli* as the bacterial screen, and it is interesting to note that Searle *et al.* (16) obtained negatives with this test. Searle *et al.* also found 2-nitro-*p*-phenylenediamine, but not 4-nitro-*o*-phenylenediamine, which is 10 times more active in the Ames test, to produce chromosome breakage in an *in vitro* test with human lymphocytes. More recently, Kirkland and Venitt (49) reported that 2-nitro-*p* and 4-nitro-*o*-phenylenediamine caused chromosome damage in cultured Chinese hamster cells, the former dye being the more active.

It was reported in April 1975 that Searle's test with mice showed two semipermanent hair colorants, containing nitro-phenylenediamines, to be carcinogenic on topical application (19). It was reported that after 64 weeks eleven mice in the test groups (164 animals) had developed lymphoid tumors while only one was observed in the control group (64 animals). However, more recent results (20) show there to be no statistical difference in tumor incidence between the control and test groups. This points up the danger of reporting the data from animal tests before completion of the test.

All the above work has received widespread press coverage with emotive headlines and has been embellished with various unsubstantiated statements by scientists in various fields. At the same time, little publicity has been given to the wealth of safety data which has been gathered by the hair dye industry over the last 10 years.

In view of the fact that all this adverse data relates to bacterial or cell culture screening procedures, it is pertinent to point out that while there is general agreement that these tests may be useful in screening large numbers of environmental materials, there is considerable scientific controversy on the correlation of the results of such tests with cancer or mutagenic risk in humans (50). Thus, Dr. Samuel Epstein (Swetland Professor of Environmental Health, Case Western Reserve University) is quoted (21) as saying of Dr. Ames' test: "Over the past 20 years about 15 of these short term tests for carcinogens have been introduced, including a few of my own. All of them have gotten a lot of publicity initially, but with the lapse of time, the reliability of each has been thrown into question. I'm not arguing with Dr. Ames' test. It's beautiful science, but I think it's being touted as doing more than it actually can."

The expert panel of the World Health Organization has concluded that "*In-vitro* mutagenicity tests alone cannot yield definitive results applicable to man" (48).

These sentiments have been expressed, by experts in the field, on numerous occasions at conferences on carcinogenesis and mutagenesis held in New York, Lyon, Ottawa, and Martinique during 1975-1976, and, on at least one occasion, in letters in scientific journals (22).

Against the results of these bacterial screening tests, it is necessary to consider the results of a number of full-scale animal studies that have shown many hair dye ingredients to be free of long-term systemic effects.

Most studies on oxidation dyes have involved topical application of freshly prepared model dye systems including addition of hydrogen peroxide. The rationale for this is based on chemical considerations and a desire to develop the most comprehensive testing method.

In hair dyeing, the user is exposed to unreacted para components and couplers as well as to reactive intermediates, particularly quinone imines, and the various indo dyes. The

oxidation of the para components by hydrogen peroxide is
relatively slow and has been shown to be incomplete even
after 24 hr. However, the coupling reactions are extremely
fast and thus there is no significant buildup in the concentration of the intermediate quinone imines. Nevertheless, it
is important that the testing protocol should involve exposure to these extremely reactive species. This cannot be
done by testing with the intermediates themselves since, in
aqueous media, they undergo rapid polymerization and/or
hydrolysis (depending on the pH) to give products that do
not arise in the oxidation dyeing process. Similarly, if
aged reaction mixtures were used, there would be little or
no exposure to the quinone imines since they are no longer
formed once the hydrogen peroxide is depleted.

The feeding of aged reaction mixtures may, at first sight,
appear to be an attractive compromise. However, under conditions prevailing in the stomach (a pH of about 2 and a
temperature of approximately 38°C), the indo dyes would undergo rapid hydrolysis to give a mixture of para components,
hydroxybenzoquinones and reaction products thereof. The
quinone products would not arise in other metabolic pathways
and the ingestion route is thus unrepresentative of the metabolism of indo dyes. Furthermore, no intermediate quinone
imines would be involved in this mode of testing. Thus,
from the chemical standpoint, topical application of fresh
reaction mixture is the only protocol involving exposure to
all the materials that are inherent in the application of
oxidation hair dyes to human subjects. This can only be
achieved by careful choice of composites, not by the use of
individual precursors in the presence of peroxide.

Four studies aimed at evaluating the carcinogenic potential of hair dye ingredients have been completed to date.
These are:

1. A study at the Battelle Institute in Frankfurt (23) involving topical application of model hair dyes to rats,
   showed no activity from 2,5-diaminotoluene, resorcinol,
   and 2,4-diaminoanisole.
2. Similar studies, sponsored by United States industry
   (24, 33), showed no effect from application of composites
   containing p-phenylenediamine, 2,5-diaminotoluene,
   resorcinol, m-phenylenediamine and 2,4-diaminoanisole to
   mice.
3. The FDA has found no effect from skin painting on mice
   with compositions containing p-phenylenediamine and
   2,5-diaminotoluene (34).
4. A 2-year skin painting study on mice, sponsored by the
   National Cancer Institute and the Eppley Institute for
   Cancer Research in Nebraska, showed no carcinogenic

effects from p-phenylenediamine and 2-nitro-4-aminophenol at the levels tested (25).

In addition to these studies, the National Cancer Institute has been sponsoring life-time feeding studies on a number of hair dye ingredients including 2,4-diaminoanisole, 2, 5-diaminotoluene, 2-nitro-p-phenylenediamine and 4-nitro-o-phenylenediamine (26). These studies which involve feeding the maximum tolerated dose of the dye in the diet, would, if negative, represent strong evidence of the noncarcinogenicity of the materials. However, it should be pointed out that these studies represent a massive exaggeration of the normal exposure to hair dyes; a positive result in such tests would not represent, a *priori*, an indication of hazard in the use of compound as an ingredient in hair coloring compositions.

Studies relevant to reproductive defects, either teratogenic or mutagenic in nature are:

1. A dominant lethal study by topical application to rats conducted by Clairol Research Laboratories, on a mixture of five dyes reported to give a positive in Ames' test, showed no evidence of mutagenic activity (27).

2. A dominant lethal study in rats, conducted by Clairol Research Laboratories, in which each of the hair dye compounds cited in Dr. Ames' paper was administered to a separate group of male animals by intraperitoneal injection, three times weekly for 8 weeks prior to mating, showed no effect (28). A similar test with 4-amino-2-nitrophenol was also negative (28).

3. A teratology study by topical application to rats, sponsored by CTFA, at the International Research Development Corporation Laboratories in Michigan showed that a large number of hair dye compounds, including all those cited by Dr. Ames, are not teratogenic (29).

4. A teratology, reproduction, and chronic toxicity study by feeding showed no effect from a group of nitrophenylenediamines and nitroaminophenols, on reproductive performance of rats and rabbits (30).

5. Dr. Bruce at the Ontario Cancer Institute, Toronto, has tested 4-nitro-o-phenylenediamine and 2,4-diaminoanisole (31) in the micronucleus and sperm abnormality assay (32) and found both compounds to be without effect.

Studies of chromosomes (16, 20) have led to the suggestion that certain hair dye ingredients, particularly semipermanent nitro dyes, might interfere with the blood-forming mechanism (20). However, a 2-year feeding study with dogs (3) and a percutaneous toxicity study in rabbits (29) indicated no abnormalities in the blood chemistry, while blood and urine analysis of a human subject reporting colored urine also revealed no abnormalities (11).

Finally, it should be mentioned that the United States hair coloring industry, through the CTFA, is continuing to support a comprehensive study of hair dye ingredients which will supplement the data discussed above with a three-generation rat reproduction study, a carcinogenicity study in rats, a carcinogenicity study in mice, and a dominant lethal study in rats for the hair dye ingredients listed in Table 3.

Again, it should be emphasized that all animal studies completed to data have shown hair dyes to be safe for their intended use. In particular, it should be noted that numerous studies relate to the materials cited by Ames *et al*. (13) and do not support his hypothesis that these materials are carcinogenic, mutagenic, or teratogenic in humans.

EPIDEMIOLOGICAL STUDIES

The article in the *New York Times* (12) makes reference to three studies alleging that hairdressers may be in special danger in respect of bladder cancer. This assertion has been traced to a scientific review (35). The only relevant quote, in this 100-page review is "The Leeds, New York and New Orleans studies all noted an excess of hairdressers and beauticians who, as indicated by Williams (1962), might have had exposure to dyestuffs."

The three studies referred to are directed toward correlation of occupation and bladder cancer incidence (36, 37, 38).

As pointed out by Menkart (39), examination of the original papers shows that they do not support the brief summary in the review, much less the strong assertions made in the newspaper articles and scientific papers (20, 49). It is interesting to compare the treatment of this subject in papers submitted before (49) and after (20) publication of the clarification (39) regarding the original papers!

The authors of the Leeds study (36) conclude "The results confirmed the risk to . . . dye workers and revealed risks to medical workers (mainly nurses), to tailors' pressers, and some groups of engineers and textile workers (associated with long-term employment only), and possibly also to hairdressers and tailors' cutters." The conclusion is speculative because the study included only five hairdressers (all male)* in a subject group of 351 cancer

---

*In Great Britain the term *hairdresser* in relation to a male includes the tradesman such as a *barber* in the U.S.

TABLE 3

List of Dyes in the Comprehensive CTFA Safety Testing Program[a]

---

p-Phenylenediamine
m-Phenylenediamine
o-Phenylenediamine
2,5-Diaminotoluene
2,4-Diaminoanisole
2,5-Diaminoanisole
2,4-Diaminophenol
p-Aminodiphenylamine
2-Amino-5-nitrophenol
2-Amino-4-nitrophenol
4-Amino-2-nitrophenol
Sodium picramate
N,N-bis(2-hydroxyethyl)-p-phenylenediamine
2,5-Diamino-4-methylanisole
5-Carbamylmethyl-amino-*o*-cresol
Resorcinol
4-Chlororesorcinol
1-Naphthol
o-Aminophenol
m-Aminophenol
p-Aminophenol
N-Methyl-*p*-aminophenol
4-Nitro-*o*-phenylenediamine
2-Nitro-*p*-phenylenediamine
Hydroquinone
Pyrogallol
2-Methylresorcinol
1,2,4-Benzenetriol
2,4,5-Toluenetriol
6-Hydroxybenzomorpholine
3-Carbamylmethylaminophenol
2-Nitro-4-bis(2-hydroxyethyl)aminodiphenylamine
2-Nitro-4-methoxydiphenylamine
2-Nitro-4'-hydroxydiphenylamine
N^4,N^4-bis(2-hydroxyethyl)-N-methyl-2-nitro-*p*-phenylenediamine
N^1,N^4,N^4-tris(2-hydroxyethyl)-2-nitro-*p*-phenylenediamine
2-Nitro-d-aminodiphenylamine
N,N-bis(2-hydroxyethyl)-2-amino-5-nitrophenol
N^1-(2-Hydroxyethyl)-4-nitro-*o*-phenylenediamine

---

[a]In addition to these hair dyes, some 34 textile dyes, used in temporary hair coloring, are being tested in the program.

patients.

The authors of the New Orleans study (38) refer to
barbers and not to hairdressers and beauticians as has been
suggested in the press. They concluded "Bladder cancer in
our study was not associated with . . . preparations for the
hair or scalp." They further noted, in respect of *barbers*
that "the comparatively small difference between numbers of
cancer and control patients (5:2) may have been due to chance
only."

Indeed the only reference to possible exposure of hairdressers to dyes is in the New York study (37) which concludes "Also under suspicion are painting, hairdressing, certain textile operations, coal mining and perhaps plumbing;
there is *possible* exposure to dyes in the first three occupations. Further data in respect of these occupations are
needed before definitive conclusions can be drawn." With regard to the reference to dyes it should be noted (i) that a
major thrust of this article is to show a connection with
occupational exposure to dye, and (ii) that the number of
hairdressers was again small--four. There is no evidence
that the hairdressers were actually questioned as to their
exposure.

It is pertinent to mention that, in a more recent study
in Massachusetts (40), the authors concluded "Although suggested by earlier studies no excess risk was found for
nurses or hairdressers."

Kirkland and Venitt (49) state that "a geographical analysis of U.S. cancer mortality based on data from 1950 to 1969
revealed excess rates for bladder and liver cancer, in men,
in counties associated with the manufacture of cosmetics."
However, they failed to point out that the study referred to
(51) also showed excess rates of one or both types of cancer
in counties associated with dyes and coal tar crudes, pharma-
ceuticals, soap and detergents, paints and varnishes, and
industrial organic chemicals. It should also have mentioned
that the counties associated with these industries show considerable, if not complete, overlap with those producing cosmetics. Furthermore, the "high incidence" counties cited by
Hoover and Fraumeri (51) are not counties associated with
the manufacture of hair dyes. Lastly, it should be noted
that the type of analysis made by Hoover and Fraumeni with
respect to cosmetics and toiletries can show correlations
which are entirely fortuitous.

Epidemiological studies are difficult and time-consuming.
However, it was reasoned that in the United States, hair dye
usage had been at such a high level for some 30 years that
any overt carcinogenicity due to hair dyes would be evident
in the total cancer mortality rates for women. The CTFA
sponsored a retrospective survey and, utilizing vital

statistics data (41), compared cancer mortality data and hair
dye usage rates over the period 1935-1972. Comparison of the
trends, even allowing for an induction period, clearly indicates there is no evidence that hair dyes have been responsible for cancer in the female population of the United States.
Indeed, while the bladder is considered the target organ for
known carcinogenic aromatic amines, the incidence rates for
bladder cancer have decreased 30% in women and increased
slightly in men over the last 30 years, during which period
the use of hair dyes has increased considerably. Even allowing for a 15-20 year induction period, any effect due to hair
dyes even at low levels of incidence would have been clearly
evident from 1965 onwards. Thus, in 1945 the use of hair
dyes by women was 5000 per 100,000 and the bladder cancer incidence rate was 8 per 100,000. In 1969 the use of hair dyes
had increased to 30,000 per 100,000 and the bladder cancer
incidence decreased to 5.2 per 100,000 (41).

Recently, based on the work of Selvin and Brown in
California, an attempt has been made to link lung cancer to
exposure to hair dyes (42). In a newspaper article (43) on
this subject, Dr. Selvin is quoted as saying, "It is difficult to understand why hair dyes should cause lung cancer
rather than, say, cancer of the scalp or the skin." It
would indeed be surprising if hair dyes were to be implicated as causative agents in lung cancer.

As to skin cancer, the CTFA posed this question to Dr.
F. Urbach, Chairman of the Skin and Cancer Hospital, Temple
University. He indicated (44) that the absence of skin
cancers in people known to be exposed to carcinogenic amines,
and the extremely low incidence of cancer of the hairy scalp
and its constancy since 1878 (about 1% of skin cancers) led
him to conclude that there is no evidence for skin cancer
being associated with the use of hair dyes. This conclusion
is further supported by the incidental observation of the
absence of effect in the skin painting studies on animals
mentioned earlier (20, 23, 24, 25, 34).

SUMMARY

Questions concerning the safety of hair dyes continue to
be based entirely on *in vitro* screening tests and unsubstantiated epidemiological speculation. In contrast, a considerable amount of safety data relating to lifetime animal
studies cannot be ignored--nor can the retrospective surveys
which show no evidence of an increase in cancer correlatable
with the level of hair dye usage.

Finally, we would mention a number of editorials in leading medical journals which support the position taken in the

present paper (45, 46, 47).

REFERENCES

1. Monnet, P. (1883). French patent 158,558.
2. Corbett, J. F. (1971). Hair Dyes. In *Chemistry of Synthetic Dyes*, ed. K. Venkataraman, Vol. 5, p. 475. New York, Academic Press.
3. Corbett, J. F. (1973). The role of meta difunctional benzene derivatives in oxidative hair dyeing: I-Reaction with p-diamines. *Soc. Cosmet. Chem. 24*: 103.
4. North American Contact Dermatitis Research Group (1972). Quoted in Ref. 5.
5. Reiss, F., and Fisher, A. A. (1974). Is hair dyed with p-phenylenediamine allergenic? *Arch. Dermatol. 109*: 221.
6. Corbett, J. F. (1969). p-Benzoquinonediimine - A vital intermediate in oxidative hair dyeing. *Soc. Cosmet. Chem. 20*:253.
7. American Medical Association (1973). Understanding hair coloring. A.M.A. Committee on Cutaneous Health and Cosmetics.
8. Lubowe, I. (1973). Allergic dermatitis and cosmetics. *Cutis 11*:431.
9. Kiese, M., and Rauscher, E. (1968). The absorption of p-toluenediamine through human skin in hair dyeing. *Toxicol. Appl. Pharmacol. 13*:325.
10. Frenkel, E. P., and Brody, F. (1973). Percutaneous absorption and elimination of an aromatic hair dye. *Arch. Environ. Health 27*:401.
10a. Maibach, H. I., Laffer, L. A., and Skinner, W. A. (1975). Percutaneous penetration following use of hair dyes. *Arch. Dermatol. 111*:1444.
11. Marshall, S., and Palmer, W. (1973). Dark urine after hair coloring. *J. Am. Med. Assoc. 226*:1010.
12. Brody, J. (1975). *New York Times*, March 18, p. 26.
13. Ames, B. N., Kammen, H. O., and Yamasaki, E. (1975). Hair dyes are mutagenic: Identification of a variety of mutagenic ingredients. *Proc. Nat. Acad. Sci. U.S.A. 72*:2423.
14. McCann, J., Choi, M., Yamasaki, E., and Ames, B. N. (1975). Detection of carcinogens as mutagens in the Salmonella/microsome test: Assay of 300 Chemicals. *Proc. Nat. Acad. Sci. U.S.A. 72*:5135.
15. McCann, J. and Ames, B. N. (1976). Detection of carcinogens as mutagens in Salmonella/microsome test: Assay of 300 chemicals: Discussion. *Proc. Nat. Acad. Sci. U.S.A. 73*:950.

16. Searle, C. E., Harnden, D. G., Venitt, S., and Gyde, O. H. B. (1975). Carcinogenicity and mutagenicity tests of some hair colorants and constituents. *Nature* *225*:506.

17. McPhee, D. G., and Podger, D. M. (1975). Hair dyes. *Med. J. Aust.* *2*:32.

18. Nishioka, H. (1975). The examination of cancer causing property of pigmented cosmetics through microbiol test, Fourth Meeting of Environmental Mutagen Society of Japan, Kyoto, Sept. 27.

19. Anonymous (1975). Another cancer link with hair dye. *New Scientist*, April 3, p. 19.

20. Venitt, S., and Searle, C. E. (1975). Mutagenicity and possible carcinogenicity of hair colorants and constituents. Meeting of the Internat. Assoc. Res. Cancer, Lyon.

21. Epstein, S. (1975). Meeting of the New York Acad. Sci., May, 1975; reported in hair dyes linked to cancer, *Med. World News* May 5, p. 31.

22. Rubin, H. (1976). Carcinogenicity tests. *Science* *191*: 241

23. Kinkel, H. J., and Holzman, S. (1973). Study of long term percutaneous toxicity and carcinogenicity of hair dyes (oxidizing dyes) in rats. *Food Cosmet. Toxicol.* *11*:641.

24. Burnett, C. M., Lanman, B., Giovaccini, R., Wolcott, G., Scala, R., and Kipplinger, M. (1975). Long term toxicity studies on oxidation hair dyes. *Good Cosmet. Toxicol.* *13*:353.

25. Shubik, P. (1975). Personal communication.

26. National Cancer Institute, Bethesda, Md. Informal communication.

27. Burnett, C. M. (1975). Personal communication.

28. Burnett, C. M., Loehr, R., and Corbett, J. F. (1977). Dominant lethal mutagenicity study on hair dyes. *J. Toxicol. Environ. Health,* Vol. 2, #3.

29. Goldenthal, E. I., Harris, S. B., Wazeter, F. X., Strausburg, J., Kapp, R., Voelker, R., and Burnett, C. M. (1976). Teratology and percutaneous toxicity studies on hair dyes. *J. Toxicol. Environ. Health*, Vol. 1, #6, p. 1027.

30. Wernick, T., Lanman, B. M., and Fraux, J. L. (1975). Chronic toxicity, teratologic, and reproduction studies with hair dyes. *Toxicol. Appl. Pharmacol. 32*:450.

31. Bruce, W. R. (1975). Personal communication.

32. Wyrobek, R. J., and Bruce, W. R. (1975). Chemical induction of sperm abnormalities in mice. *Proc. Nat. Acad. Sci. U.S.A. 72*:4425.

33. Fraux, J. L. (1973). Personal communication.

34. Giles, A. L., Chung, C. W., and Kommineni, C. (1976). Dermal carcinogenicity study by mouse-skin painting with 2,4-diaminotoluene alone or in representative hair dye formulations. *J. Toxicol. Environ. Health* *1*:433.

35. Clayson, D. B., and Cooper, E. H. (1970). Cancer of the urinary tract. *Adv. Cancer Res.* *13*:271.

36. Anthony, H. M., and Thomas, G. M. (1970). Tumors of the urinary bladder: An analysis of the occupations of 1,030 patients in Leeds, England. *J. Nat. Cancer Inst.* *45*:879.

37. Wynder, E. L., Onerdonk, J., and Mantel, N. (1963). An epidemiological investigation of cancer of the bladder. *Cancer* *16*:1388.

38. Durham, L. T., Rabson, A. S., Steward, H. L., Frank, A. S., and Young, J. L. (1968). Rates, interview, and pathology study of cancer of the urinary bladder in New Orleans, La. *J. Nat. Cancer Inst.* *41*:683.

39. Menkart, J. (1975). Excess bladder cancer in beauticians? *Science* *190*:96.

40. Cole, P., Hoover, R., and Friedell, C. H. (1972). Occupation and cancer of the lower urinary tract. *Cancer* *29*:1250.

41. U. S. Public Health Service. Vital Statistics of the United States. Annual Reports. Washington, D.C., U.S. Government Printing Office.

42. Selvin, S., and Brown, S. M. (1975). Quoted by P. Toynbee and N. Hawkes, *London Observer*, July 13, p. 1.

43. Hawkes, N., and Toynbee, P. (1975). *Sunday Observer*, July 13.

44. Urbach, F. (1973). Personal communication to C. M. Burnett.

45. Editorial (1975). Hair dyes and cancer, *Lancet* *2*:218.

46. Editorial (1975). Facile mutagenesis by hair dye constituents. *Br. Med. J.* *4*:188.

47. Editorial (1975). Cancer! Alarm! Cancer! *New Engl. J. Med.* *293*:1319.

Controlling Infections:
The Hospital Environment and Handwashing

George F. Mallison and Allen C. Steere, Jr.

Bacterial Disease Division, Center for Disease Control
Atlanta, Georgia
and
Yale-New Haven Hospital
New Haven, Connecticut

The Center for Disease Control (CDC) has been conducting investigations on the epidemiology and control of nosocomial (hospital-acquired) disease for more than 10 years. As a result of these studies, some general characteristics of nosocomial infections in hospitals have become apparent. On the average, about 5% of individuals admitted to short-term, general hospitals will acquire an infection as a result of their hospital stay (1, 2). Rates of infections associated with hospitalization vary with hospitals; however, higher rates are often associated with large teaching hospitals, and lower rates may be associated with small community hospitals (1). If the same definitions for infections that result in the 5% average rate of nosocomial infections are used for surveillance for community-acquired infections, about 10% of individuals will be found to have infections on admission to the hospital (2).

The proportion of nosocomial infections that might be prevented by active programs in hospitals is not known; CDC now has underway some detailed studies to evaluate more clearly the preventability of infections in hospitals (3). Until data from these studies are available, our current estimates are that perhaps half of the infections acquired in hospitals might not occur in the presence of highly effective hospital programs for prevention. It is our opinion that prompt and adequate handwashing is the single most

important measure to reduce preventable infections in hospitals (4). The importance of handwashing in control of
nosocomial infections was recognized by Semmelweiss over
100 years ago (5). Infections thought to be transferred by
contaminated hands of patient-care personnel have been discussed in a large number of published papers discussing a
number of sites of infection and a number of locations within hospitals (6-18).

The Center for Disease Control and the American Hospital
Association have recommended that personnel wash their hands
before and after taking care of each patient (4, 19). But
it is widely known that personnel in hospitals do not wash
their hands consistently before and after patient contacts.
Realistically, the risk of transmitting organisms to a given
patient or acquiring organisms from a given patient varies
with the type of contact with the patient, as well as a number of other factors. It is extremely difficult to motivate
all members of the hospital staff to wash their hands frequently during patient-care activities. Handwashing itself
may be a cause of hospital disease (dermatitis) among hospital staff members if conducted too frequently or with the
use of products that might be irritating to the skin.

Thus, it is commonly observed in hospitals that personnel
do not wash their hands when they should and as frequently as
they should. Yet, the principal disagreement among hospital
personnel generally involves which agent or agents should be
used as an aid to handwashing. Many have believed that antiseptic agents (products used on the skin to kill microorganisms) should be used for all handwashing by patient-care
personnel. Others believe that antiseptic agents should be
reserved only for special purposes and that for routine
handwashing, plain soap (or detergent) preparations should
be used because, although such preparations do not kill many
organisms, they suspend microbial contamination so that it
may be removed easily from the skin under running water. A
survey conducted in 1974 of 82 hospitals in CDC's National
Nosocomial Infection Study showed that somewhat over half of
these hospitals required handwashing with an antiseptic between all patient contacts; the antiseptic recommended most
frequently was an iodophor-type product. Slightly less than
half the hospitals surveyed required handwashing solely with
plain soap between routine patient contacts.

Many studies on handwashing have used only a comparison
of counts of microorganisms on the hands before and after a
single handwash as the criterion for effectiveness of the
agent (20-25). Most studies have not evaluated the effects
of frequent handwashing over a longer period of time on
bacterial flora of the hands or on dermatitis of the hands;
this latter factor has, in our experience, been influential

in the actual acceptance and use of particular handwashing products in hospitals.

RESIDENT AND TRANSIENT MICROBIAL FLORA

In describing the microbial flora on the hands, most investigators discuss "resident" and "transient" microbial flora (24). Resident flora are generally described as organisms that survive and multiply on or in the skin and, thus, can be found repeatedly from cultures of an individual person. Transient flora are described as organisms that do not survive and multiply on or in the skin and, thus, are easily removable and cannot be cultured repeatedly from a particular individual. Almost everyone has aerobic staphylococci and diphtheroids as resident flora on most skin areas (26, 27). Gram-positive organisms are much more common on the skin than gram-negative ones (28). The hair, face, axilla, and the groin usually have the greatest number of microorganisms, while the arms and hands generally have the fewest (29). On the hands, the greatest number of organisms readily available for sampling generally are found around and under the fingernails (26).

"Resident" skin flora are usually of low virulence, and they rarely cause infections other than skin infections. However, they may cause infections when introduced into the body through invasive procedures such as surgery or catheterization. Resident organisms on the skin are not easily removed by scrubbing, but they can be inactivated by antiseptic agents (24).

Transient microbial flora may consist of a large variety of pathogenic organisms, including all those that commonly cause nosocomial infections. When applied to the skin, these organisms generally survive less than 24 hr (30). It is apparent that transient flora are readily removable, quickly and effectively, by handwashing with soap and water for 15 seconds or so; an antiseptic does not seem to be necessary for such removal, and the use of friction between the hands and running water alone may be almost as effective as the use of soap and water in removing transient organisms (31, 32).

Organisms such as *Staphylococcus aureus* and a number of gram-negatives can be *either* resident *or* transient flora. More commonly, *S. aureus* is a resident organism in either the interior nares or the perineum; less commonly it resides on the hands (33-37). In persons with exezematous or dermatitic skin, *S. aureus* and gram-negative organisms frequently colonize the diseased skin (38). Resident carriage of gram-negative organisms on the hands has been reported in nursery

personnel (39). However, it remains unclear whether such
carriage of gram-negative organisms occurs because of repeated exposure to them or because frequent use of antiseptics encourages colonization.

The purpose of most handwashing in patient care should
be simply to remove transient microbial contamination that
has been acquired by recent contact with people or objects.
The risk of acquisition of microbial contamination of the
hands varies with the type of contact. Patient-care personnel who have contact with patient excretions, secretions, or
blood, either directly or through contaminated objects, may
acquire carriage of microorganisms from such contact. Examination of a patient's mouth, nose, vagina, urethra, or
rectum may cause contamination of the hands. Transient contamination of the hands also may occur from contact of contaminated items such as bedpans, urinals, urine bags, and
sheets or dressings of patients.

The majority of patient-care involves generally minimal
contact with the patient (40). Nurses and aides have more
direct, personal contact with patients than physicians. We
believe that the risk of causing infections or even acquiring organisms from patients is probably minimal with activities such as shaking hands, taking the pulse or oral temperature, listening to the heart or percussing the chest,
palpating the abdomen, or administering medications.

The patients who are most likely to acquire infections
because of "dirty" hands are those with catheters and other
invasive devices, including a majority of patients in
intensive-care units, those with depressed host resistance,
and newborn infants (6-18).

DESCRIPTION OF HANDWASHING AGENTS

Soaps and Detergents

These products come in many forms: bar, liquid, granule,
leaflet, or soap-impregnated tissues. All have been found
acceptable by patient-care personnel; however, contaminated
liquid soap dispensers have been associated with nosocomial
outbreaks (41-44). Such dispensers should be emptied,
cleaned, and refilled regularly. To our knowledge, no disease outbreaks have been caused by contaminated bar soap;
however, bars of soap frequently remain wet and could support the growth of organisms; therefore, small bars that can
be replaced frequently should be used, and soap bars should
be placed on racks that allow drainage of water.

Many hospitals have chosen a form of soap that remains
dry before use because of problems that may be associated

with liquid soap or wet bars of soap. Soap leaflets or soap-impregnated paper tissues are dry before use, and they also have the advantage of requiring about 15 seconds of hand-washing once the procedure is begun because that period of time is necessary to permit lathering and rinsing.

Alcohol

Alcohol has been used as an antiseptic for many years, and it is still one of the most effective products available. Handwashing with ethyl or isopropyl alcohol for 1 to 3 minutes will reduce bacterial counts on the hands by 90% or more (22, 23). However, alcohol is volatile and flammable, it evaporates quickly, and it dries the skin unless it is mixed with emollients.

Iodine

Iodine, like alcohol, is an effective antiseptic agent that has been used for many years. Iodine kills vegatative organisms, spores, viruses, and fungi. The combination of iodine and alcohol to form a tincture (approximately 2 grams per 100 milliliters of approximately 50% alcohol) is a most effective antiseptic (43-47). However, tincture of iodine may cause burning, chapping, and allergic reactions; this preparation is generally used only as a skin antiseptic prior to a hypodermic injection or an operative incision rather than for routine handwashing (43).

Iodophors

The iodophors are water-soluble complexes of iodine in which the iodine is bound and released more slowly than with a tincture, thereby reducing the problems of adverse skin reactions and staining caused by tincture of iodine. Approximately 60 to 90% reduction of the microorganism count on hands can result from 2 minutes of handwashing with iodophors (21, 48). However, the U.S. Food and Drug Administration (FDA) recently purlished a warning about the effectiveness and safety of iodophors (49). In our experience, many hospital infection control personnel have found iodophor preparations to be considerably more drying to the skin than other antiseptic handwashing agents if used frequently for handwashing.

Hexachlorophene Preparations

Antiseptics containing hexachlorophene (HCP), if used at least daily for at least 3 to 5 days, are approximately

as effective as iodophors in reducing resident skin flora
(21, 45, 50). HCP has a substantive (binding to the stratum
corneum) effect, reducing the number of inoculated S. aureus
able to survive on the skin (29, 51). Bathing infants with
HCP has been shown to be effective in reducing the incidence
of S. aureus infections (52), but three study reports have
indicated that routine handwashing with HCP by nursery personnel did not reduce infections in newborn infants (38, 53,
54). No difference was found between rates of S. aureus
surgical wound infections in groups cared for by personnel
who washed their hands with HCP versus groups who washed
their hands with soap and water (55). Heavy use of HCP has
been associated with blood hexichlorophene levels, but the
long-term effects of such levels are not known at present
(56). HCP preparations have minimal activity against gram-
negative bacteria and fungi, and may even enhance their
growth (38, 53, 57, 58). More gram-negative contamination
of hands has been found when HCP antiseptics are used than
when soap and water or iodophor and water are used (39, 59).
However, in 36 nurseries surveyed by CDC in 1972, infants
bathed with HCP did not have a higher incidence of gram-
negative infections than infants bathed with soap and water
(57).

Chlorhexidine

The British have had considerable experience with
chlorhexidine-containing products. Such products may be
approximately as effective as iodophors or hexachlorophene
in reducing resident flora (50). Products containing
chlorhexidine will probably be permitted for sale by the
FDA in the United States in the near future.

Aqueous Benzalkonium or Benzethonium Chloride Products

These products have been used as handwashing agents,
but they are relatively ineffective; in addition, they are
rapidly inactivated by organic materials, and contamination
with pathogenic gram-negative organisms has occurred (60-66).

Antiseptic Foams

Because handwashing sinks sometimes may not be conveniently located, antiseptic foams have been developed for use
either at the bedside of patients or to be carried with personnel for use when needed when a sink with running water is
not available for handwashing. About 10 years ago a product
containing emollients, quaternary ammonium compounds, and
alcohol was commercially available in the United States; at

this writing two new foam products, with alcohol and with alcohol-HCP, are commercially available. Such products are useful when it is not realistically possible to provide proper handwashing facilities.

HANDWASHING RECOMMENDATIONS

From the information above on skin flora and on handwashing agents, we believe that adequate handwashing for hospital personnel should include handwashing with antiseptic agents before doing surgery or certain other invasive procedures such as catheterization and in isolation rooms; but handwashing with only soap and water is recommended between more routine patient contacts.

A policy such as this has been criticized because some patient-care personnel may be carriers of pathogenic organisms as part of their resident hand flora. And, further, antiseptics may have a sustained action to suppress skin flora, so antiseptic handwashing might be desirable. We disagree with this criticism, however, because all currently available antiseptics have some adverse effects (67). Even those that may ordinarily be safe can cause excessive dryness, cracking, and dermatitis with repeated use. If this were to occur, antiseptics used continuously might do more harm than good, because bacterial counts on dermatitic skin cannot be reduced appreciably even with antiseptics (59, 68, 69, 70). Colonization with *S. aureus* and gram-negative organisms may become more common (38, 71). Personnel with dermatitic hands may tend to avoid handwashing altogether. In some persons, even frequent handwashing with soap and water without antiseptics can cause the skin to become excessively dry; however, reports we have received suggest that dermatitis occurs most frequently with antiseptics, particularly those containing iodophors. Thus, CDC favors a handwashing policy that reserves the use of antiseptics for special situations where the risk of infection is greatest; we recommend handwashing solely with soap and water for routine patient care.

Handwashing in Patient-Care Areas

Handwashing procedures themselves are simple. The hands should be vigorously lathered and rubbed together for at least 15 seconds under a moderate-size stream of comfortably warm water. Then the hands should be rinsed and dried with a paper towel, and the towel then used to turn off the faucet. This handwashing procedure should always be used unless it is absolutely impossible to conveniently get to a source of running water for handwashing.

Cracked or chipped nail polish or rings on the fingers make the removal of organisms from hands more difficult (72). Therefore, we recommend that patient-care personnel not wear rings or nail polish while on duty; however, many hospitals permit personnel to wear a single wedding band.

Personnel who have contact with patient excretions, secretions, or blood should wash their hands with soap and water after each such contact. This should avoid contamination of the employee or of persons or objects that a person might subsequently contact. However, the CDC manual, "Isolation Techniques for Use in Hospitals," recommends that antiseptic agents be used after contact with secretions or excretions from isolated patients (4). Antiseptic handwashing is also recommended before changing dressings on infected wounds (4).

Personnel should wash their hands with soap and water before inserting or caring for intravenous, urinary, or peritoneal catheters or other invasive devices. Patients with such devices or catheters are at risk of acquisition of nosocomial infections because of carriage of pathogenic organisms on the hands of personnel caring for their devices. Gloves are usually worn before the insertion of catheters, and CDC recommends their use to minimize the risk of personnel causing infections in patients. However, gloves often are not worn before the insertion of intravenous catheters in hospitals in spite of our recommendations. Therefore, handwashing with an antiseptic agent, preferably an iodophor, is recommended as a minimal precaution before this procedure, since resident flora on the hands of personnel may cause infections at intravenous sites.

Personnel should wash their hands before activities that require touching either a large skin area or mucous membranes. Handwashing should not be necessary before patient care activities with minimal contact, such as shaking hands, taking a pulse or an oral temperature, palpating the abdomen, listening to the heart or percussing the chest, or giving medications. However, if gross contamination occurs during such generally minimal patient-contact activities, handwashing is definitely indicated immediately thereafter.

Although personnel should be able to identify procedures and patients that might be associated with the greatest risk of infection, they generally do not know if they have acquired hand carriage of pathogens, and they cannot always readily and quickly identify patients with invasive devices that might make the risk of acquisition of infection more likely. Furthermore, although personnel may expect when they begin a patient-care activity to have only minimal contact with the patient, unexpected activities may require

handling of devices or extensive contact. *Thus, we believe
that the discipline of washing one's hands before "hands-on"
care of all patients is to be encouraged.*

Intensive Care Unit

Because of the high susceptibility to infection of many
patients in intensive care units, personnel in these units
should wash their hands more often than personnel in many
other areas. Handwashing with soap and water should suffice
before (and/or after) most contacts, although antiseptic
agents should be available for handwashing before certain
invasive procedures.

Nursery

Because of the high susceptibility of newborns to skin
infections, handwashing between infant contacts is particularly important to help prevent infection. At the time of
the widespread discontinuation of hexachlorophene (HCP)
bathing of infants in 1971, the FDA and the American Academy
of Pediatrics recommended that nursery personnel wash their
hands either with an iodophor or an antiseptic containing
3% HCP between infant contacts and for 2 minutes at the beginning of each working day (67, 73). Unfortunately, there
are few data to suggest that antiseptic handwashing is of
greater benefit than soap and water handwashing in the
nursery (38, 53, 54). We would like to encourage research-
ers who study the effects of iodophors and HCP preparations
for handwashing in the nursery also to study the effects of
soap control.

Personnel with Dermatitis

If personnel have dermatitis because of frequent handwashing, they may be of greater risk to patients. As was
indicated above, colonization of dermatitic skin with viru-
lent organisms is common, handwashing does not appreciably
reduce bacterial counts under these conditions, and personnel with dermatitis may tend to avoid handwashing. Once an
employee problem of dermatitis has begun, the use of hand
creams, alternating the handwashing agent used, or wearing
gloves may help alleviate the problem. However, hand creams
are not necessarily sterile, and therefore it would be preferable that they be applied only after handwashing away
from duty. If indicated for use during patient-care activities, the hand creams should be sterile and should be fur-
nished in small containers that will be used up quickly. If
personnel with dermatitis wear gloves during duty, they will

be protected from handwashing agents and patients will be
protected by the gloves. The gloved hands should be
washed (or gloves should be changed) as frequently as hands
would be washed if gloves were not worn. Microbial contamination is washed away more easily from gloves than from
nongloved hands (31). However, if dermatitis persists, em-
ployees should report either to the hospital employee health
service or to their physician for evaluation and treatment.

Surgical, Obstetric, and Major Catheterization Procedures

Surgical and obstetric procedures require the highest
consistency and degree of hand asepsis, because these procedures may be prolonged and both the resident and transient
flora of the hands could be introduced into wounds from
hands of personnel. Gloves are commonly worn for such procedures, and bacteria grow faster under gloves than on un-
gloved hands (24). Hand asepsis becomes important because
gloves may puncture or tear; a number of studies have reported 5 to 60% of operations accompanied by glove punctures (70, 74, 75). Glove punctures are often associated
with handling suture needles with a gloved hand rather than
with forceps, handling wire sutures, or touching sharp
edges of bone. Cruse and Foord reported that the clean
wound infection rate in their hospital was 3 times higher
after operations that were accompanied by glove tears than
those that were not known to have been accompanied by glove
tears (76).

Surgical hand scrubs should begin by cleaning the fingernails with a plastic or orangewood stick. After this, the
hands should be scrubbed for 4 to 5 minutes either with an
iodophor or a HCP antiseptic (77, 78). Scrubbing with 70%
alcohol also has been used (68, 77). An iodophor has the
advantage of its broad antibacterial effect; however, HCP,
because of its substantive (binding) effect, may allow a
longer period of time with low bacterial counts on the skin
under gloves (48). Cruse and Foord found no difference in
clean wound infection rates in patients when an iodophor or
a hexachlorophene-containing preparation was used for surgical scrub (76). Scrubbing with a sterile brush seems to
offer no advantage over scrubbing with a sterile sponge in
reducing bacterial counts (79, 80). Tap water is rarely
sterile; therefore, any small possibilities of microbial
contamination of orangewood sticks or brushes or sponges
used in scrubbing should not cause any great concern.

SUMMARY

Hospital personnel should wash their hands before and after any significant contact with any patient. The risk of personnel acquiring transient hand-carriage of organisms is usually greatest after contact with excretions, secretions, or blood; patients at greatest risk are those undergoing surgery, those with catheters, and newborn infants. Although handwashing with an antiseptic agent between patient contacts is theoretically desirable, handwashing with soap, running water, and mechanical friction is sufficient to remove most transiently acquired organisms. Many antiseptic agents product excessively dry skin if used frequently, and any regimen of handwashing that leads to dermatitis may negate the purpose of handwashing. We favor antiseptics for handwashing before surgery and other high-risk invasive procedures, in the care of newborn infants, and in handwashing for isolated patients; but generally we recommend soap and water for other handwashing.

REFERENCES

1. Bennett, J. V., Scheckler, W. E., Maki, D. G., and Brachman, P. S. August 3-6, 1970. Current national patterns, United States. Proceedings of the International Conference on Nosocomial Infections. Center for Disease Control, ed. P. S. Brachman and T. C. Eickhoff.
2. Scheckler, W. E., Garner, J. S., Kaiser, A. B., and Bennett, J. V. August 3-6, 1970. Prevalence of infections and antibiotic usage in eight community hospitals. Proceedings of the International Conference on Nosocomial Infections, Center for Disease Control. Edited by P. S. Brachman and T. C. Eickhoff.
3. Anonymous. (1975). Survey of infection control programs to be undertaken. *Hospitals* *49*:71.
4. Center for Disease Control (1975). Isolation techniques for use in hospitals, 2nd edition. Washington, D. C., U.S. Government Printing Office.
5. Semmelweiss, I. P. (1861). Die Actiologie, der Begriff und die Prophylaxis des Kindbettfiebers.
6. Selden, R., Lee, S., Wang, W. L. L., Bennett, J. V., and Eickhoff, T. C. (1971). Nosocomial klebsiella infections: Intestinal colonization as a reservoir. *Ann. Intern. Med.* 74:657.
7. Salzman, T. C., Clark, J. J., and Klemm, L. (1967). Hand contamination of personnel as a mechanism of cross-infection in nosocomial infections with antibiotic-

resistant *E. coli* and *Klebsiella aerobacter*. *Antimi-crob. Agents Chemother.* p. 97.

8. Adler, J. L., Burke, J. P., Martin, D. F., and Finland, M. (1971). Proteus infections in a general hospital. II. Some clinical and epidemiological characteristics. With an analysis of 71 cases of proteus bacteremia. *Ann. Intern. Med.* *75*:531.

9. Lowbury, E. J. L., Thom, B. T., Lilly, H. A., Babb, J. H., and Whittall, K. (1970). Sources of infection with *Pseudomonas aeruginosa* in patients with tracheostomy. *J. Med. Microbiol.* *3*:39.

10. Rammelkamp, C. H., Jr., Mortimer, E. A., Jr. and Wolinsky, E. (1964). Transmission of streptococcal and staphylococcal infections. *Ann. Intern. Med.* *60*:753.

11. Mortimer, E. A., Jr., Lipsitz, P. J., Wolinsky, E., Gonzaga, A. J., and Rammelkamp, C, H., Jr. (1962). Transmission of staphylococci between newborns: Importance of the hands of personnel. *Am. J. Dis. Child.* *104*:289.

12. Mortimer, E. A., Jr., Wolinsky, E., Gonzaga, A. J., and Rammelkamp, C. H., Jr. (1966). Role of airborne transmission in staphylococcal infections. *Br. Med. J.* *1*: 319.

13. Frappier-Davignon, L., Frappier, A., and St. Pierre, J. (1959). Staphylococcal infection in hospital nurseries. Influence of three different nursing techniques. *Can. Med. Assoc. J.* *81*:531.

14. Fleck, A. C., Jr., and Klein, J. O. (1959). The epidemiology and investigation of hospital-acquired staphylococcal disease in newborn infants. *Pediatrics* *24*:1102.

15. Wolinsky, E., Lipsitz, P. J., Mortimer, E. A., Jr., and Rammelkamp, C. H., Jr. (1960). Acquisition of staphylococci by newborns. Direct versus indirect transmission. *Lancet* *2*:620.

16. Eisenach, K. D., Reber, R. M., Eitzman, D. B., and Baer, H. (1972). Nosocomial infections due to hanamycin-resistant [R]-factor carrying enteric organisms in an intensive care nursery. *Pediatrics* *50*:395.

17. Adler, J. L., Schulman, J. A., Terry, P. M., Feldman, D. B., and Skally, P. (1970). Nosocomial colonization with kanamycin-resistant *Klebsiella pneumoniae*, types 2 and 11, in a premature nursery. *J. Pediatr.* *77*:376.

18. Burke, J. P., Ingall, D., Klein, J. O., Gezon, H. M., and Finland, M. (1971). Proteus mirabilis infections in a hospital nursery traced to a human carrier. *N. Engl. J. Med.* *284*:115.

19. American Hospital Association (1974). Infection control in the hospital, 3rd edition, p. 111. Chicago.
20. Dineen, P. (1971). Clinical research in skin disinfection. *Assoc. Operat. Room Nurses J. 14*:73.
21. Lowbury, E. J. L., Lilly, H. A., and Bull, J. P. (1963). Disinfection of hands: Removal of resident bacteria. *Br. Med. J. 1*:1251.
22. Gardner, A. D., and Seddon, J. H. (1946). Rapid chemical disinfection of clean unwashed skin. *Lancet 1*:683.
23. Dineen, P., and Hildick-Smith, G. (1965). Antiseptic care of the hands. In *Skin Bacteria and Their Role in Infections*, ed. H. I. Maibach and G. Hildick-Smith, p. 29. New York, McGraw-Hill.
24. Price, P. B. (1938). New studies in surgical bacteriology and surgical technique. *J. Am. Med. Assoc. 111*: 1993.
25. Gibbs, B. M., and Stuttard, L. W. (1967). Evaluation of skin germicides. *J. Appl. Bacteriol. 30*:66.
26. Kligman, A. M. (1965). The bacteriology of normal skin. In *Skin Bacteria and Their Role in Infection*, ed. H. I. Maibach, and G. Hildick-Smith, p. 16. New York, McGraw-Hill.
27. Marples, M. J. (1969). The normal flora of the human skin. *Br. J. Dermatol. 81*(Suppl):15.
28. Marples, M. J. (1969). Life on the human skin. *Sci. Am. 218*:108.
29. Marples, M. J. (1969). The normal flora of the human skin. *Br. J. Dermatol. 81*(Suppl):2.
30. Blank, I. H. (1965). Survival of bacteria on the skin. In *Skin Bacteria and Their Role in Infection*, ed. H. I. Maibach, and G. Hildick-Smith, p. 46. New York, McGraw-Hill.
31. Lowbury, E. J. L., Lilly, H. A., and Bull, J. P. (1964). Disinfection of hands: Removal of transient organisms. *Br. Med. J. 2*:230.
32. Sprunt, K., Redman, W., and Leidy, G. (1973). Antibacterial effectiveness of routine handwashing. *Pediatrics 52*:264.
33. Williams, R. E. O. (1965). Pathogenic bacterial on the skin. In *Skin Bacteria and Their Role in Infection*, ed. H. I. Maibach, and G. Hildick-Smith, p. 50. New York, McGraw-Hill.
34. Williams, R. E. O. (1963). Healthy carriage of Staphylococcus aureus: Its prevalence and importance. *Bacteriol. Rev. 27*:56.
35. Williams, R. E. O. (1965). Pathogenic bacteria on the skin. In *Skin Bacteria and Their Role in Infection*, ed. H. I. Maibach, and G. Hildick-Smith, p. 54. New York, McGraw-Hill.

36. Nahmias, A. J., and Eickhoff, T. C. (1964). Staphylo-
    coccal infections in hospitals. *N. Engl. J. Med. 265*:
    74, 120, 177.
37. Hare, R., and Ridley, M. (1958). Transmission of Staph
    aureus. *Br. Med. J. 1*:69.
38. Forfar, J. O., Gould, J. C., and Maccabe, A. F. (1968).
    Effect of hexachlorophene on incidence of staphylococcal
    and gram-negative infection in the newborn. *Lancet 2*:
    177.
39. Knittle, M. A., Eitzman, D. V., and Baer, H. (1975).
    Role of hand contamination of personnel in the epi-
    demiology of gram-negative nosocomial infections.
    J. Pediatr. 86:433.
40. Fox, M. K., Langner, S. B., and Well, R. W. (1974).
    How good are handwashing practices? *Am. J. Nurs. 74*:
    1676.
41. National Nosocomial Infections Study Quarterly Report,
    Second Quarter 1972 (1974). Serratia marcescens in an
    intensive care unit. Atlanta, Center for Disease
    Control, p. 9.
42. Lowbury, E. J. L. (1951). Contamination of cetrimide
    and other fluids with *Pseudomonas pyocyanea*. *Br. J.
    Ind. Med. 8*:22.
43. U.S. General Services Administration (1974). O-T-C
    topical antimicrobial products and drug and cosmetic
    products. *Fed. Regist. 39*(179), part 2:33116.
44. Spaulding, E. H. (1971). Role of chemical disinfection
    in the prevention of nosocomial infections. Proceedings
    of the International Conference on Nosocomial Infec-
    tions, Center for Disease Control, Edited by
    P. S. Brachman, and T. C. Eickhoff, p. 247.
45. Price, P. B. (1968). Surgical antiseptics. In
    Disinfection, Sterilization, and Preservation, ed.
    C. A. Lawrence, and S. S. Black, p. 532. Philadelphia,
    Lea & Febiger.
46. White, J. J., Wallace, C. K., and Burnett, L. S. (1970).
    Skin disinfection. *Johns Hopkins Med. J. 126*:169.
47. Gershenfeld, L. (1968). Iodine. In *Disinfection,
    Sterilization, and Preservation*, ed. C. A. Lawrence,
    and S. S. Black, p. 329. Philadelphia, Lea & Febiger.
48. Michaud, R. N., McGrath, M. D., and Goss, W. A. (1974).
    Multi-parameter measurements of skin-degerming activity
    on the hand (abstract). Chicago, 74th Annual Meeting
    of the Society of Microbiology.
49. U.S. General Services Administration (1974). O-T-C
    topical antimicrobial products and drug and cosmetic
    products. *Fed. Regist. 39*(179) part 2:33131.
50. Lilly, H. A., and Lowbury, E. J. L. (1971). Disinfec-
    tion of the skin: An assessment of some new prepara-
    tions. *Br. Med. J. 3*:674.

51. Von Der Hoeven, E., and Hinton, N. A. (1968). An assessment of the prolonged effect of antiseptic scrubs on the bacterial flora of the hands. *Can. Med. Assoc. J. 99*:402.

52. Kaslow, R. A., Dixon, R. E., Martin, S. M., Mallison, C. F., Goldman, D. A., Lindsey, J. D., II, Rhame, F. S., and Bennett, J. V. (1973). Staphylococcal disease related to hospital nursery bathing practices - a nationwide epidemiologic investigation. *Pediatrics 51*:418.

53. Light, I. J., Sutherland, J. M., Cochran, L., and Sutorius, J. (1968). Ecologic relation between *Staphylococcus aureus* and *pseudomonas* in a nursery population. *N. Engl. J. Med. 278*:1243.

54. Mortimer, E. A., Jr., Wolinsky, E., and Rammelkamp, C, H., Jr. (1965). The transmission of staphylococci by the hands of personnel. In *Skin Bacteria and Their Role in Infection,* ed. H. I, Maibach, and G. Hildick-Smith, p. 187. New York, McGraw-Hill.

55. Bruun, J. N. (1970). Post operative wound infection. *Acta Med. Scand.* [Suppl.]*514*:33.

56. U.S. General Services Administration (1974). O-T-C topical antimicrobial products and drug and cosmetic products. *Fed. Regist. 39*(179), part 2:33118.

57. National Nosocomial Infections Study Quarterly Report, Fourth Quarter 1972 (1974). Nosocomial infections in nurseries and their relationship to hospital infant bathing practices - a preliminary report. Atlanta, Center for Disease Control, p. 9.

58. Miller, J. M., Jackson, D. A., and Collier, C. S. (1962). The microbial property of pHisoHex. *Milit. Med. 127*:576.

59. Bruun, J. N., and Solberg, C. O. (1973). Hand carriage of gram-negative bacilli and staphylococcus aureus. *Br. Med. J. 2*:580.

60. Adair, F. W., Geftic, S. G., and Gelzer, J. (1969). Resistance of pseudomonas to quaternary ammonium compounds. I. Growth in benzalkonium chloride solution. *Appl. Microbiol. 18*:299.

61. Adair, F. W., Geftic, S. G., and Gelzer, J. (1971). Resistance of pseudomanas to quaternary ammonium compounds. *Appl. Microbiol. 21*:1058.

62. Chaplin, C. E. (1952). Bacterial resistance to quaternary ammonium compounds. *J. Bacteriol. 63*:453.

63. Lee, J. C., and Fiaklow, P. J. (1961). Benzalkonium chloride - source of hospital infection with gram-negative bacteria. *J. Am. Med. Assoc. 177*:708.

64. U.S. General Services Administration (1974). O-T-C topical antimicrobial products and drug and cosmetic products. *Fed. Regist. 39*(179), part 2:33131.

65. Plotkin, S. A., and Austrian, R. (1958). Bacteremia caused by *Pseudomonas* spp. following the use of material stored in solutions of a cationic surface-active agent. *Am. J. Med. Sci.* *235*:621.

66. Malizia, W. F., Gangarosa, E. J., and Goley, A. F. (1960). Benzalkonium chloride as a source of infection. *N. Engl. J. Med.* *263*:800.

67. U.S. General Services Administration (1974). O-T-C topical antimicrobial products and drug and cosmetic products. *Fed. Regist.* *39*(179), part 2:33102.

68. Price, P. B. (1960). Skin antisepsis. In *Lectures in Sterilization*, ed. J. H. Brewer, p. 79. Durham, North Carolina, Duke University Press.

69. Walter, C. W. (1965). Disinfection of hands. *Am. J. Surg.* *109*:691.

70. Walter, C. W., and Kundsin, R. B. (1969). The bacteriologic study of surgical gloves from 250 operations. *Surg. Gynecol. Obstet.* *129*:949.

71. Kligman, A. M. (1965). The bacteriology of normal skin. In *Skin Bacteria and Their Role in Infection*, ed. H. I. Maibach, and G. Hildick-Smith, p. 26. New York, McGraw-Hill.

72. The sub-committee on aseptic methods in operating theatres of the committee on hospital infection: Aseptic methods in the operating suite (1968). *Lancet* *1*:706.

73. Hexachlorophene in newborns. *FDA Drug Bull.* December 1971. Copies may be obtained from the Bureau of Drugs, FDA, Washington, D. C.

74. Shouldice, E. E., and Martin, C. J. (1959). Wound infections, surgical gloves and hands of operating personnel. *Can. Med. Assoc. J.* *81*:636.

75. Lowbury, E. J. L., and Lilly, H. A. (1960). Disinfection of hands of surgeons and nurses. *Br. Med. J.* *1*:1445.

76. Cruse, P. J. E., and Foord, R. (1973). A five-year prospective study of 23,649 surgical wounds. *Arch. Surg.* *107*:206.

77. Dineen, P. (1970). Prevention of infection in the operating room. *Bull. Am. Coll. Surg.* *55*:18.

78. Povidone-iodine (Betadine) for surgical antisepsis (1969). *Med. Lett.* *11*:99.

79. Bornside, G. H., Crowder, V. H., and Cohn, I. (1968). A bacteriological evaluation of surgical scrubbing with disposable iodophor-soap impregnated polyurethane scrub sponges. *Surgery* *64*:743.

80. Michaud, R. N., McGrath, B. M., and Goss, W. A. (1972). Improved experimental model for measuring skin degerming activity on the human hand. *Antimicrob. Agents Chemother.* *2*:8.

The Cutaneous Absorption
and Systemic Toxicity of Antimicrobials:
FDA Concerns

Mary K. Bruch

Division of Anti-Infective Drug Products
Bureau of Drugs
Food and Drug Administration
Rockville, Maryland

My purpose is to share with you the lessons learned in the exposition of hexachlorophene toxicity and the present concerns of FDA in the review of topically applied products. This level of interest and public attention to an issue has seldom been equaled; it is present to such an extent that Peter Benchley in *Jaws* refers to youthful lack of involvement by noting several issues, including the finding that hexachlorophene caused brain damage, which seemed not to touch them.

The events of the last few years have irrevocably changed the way in which topical products, and antimicrobial products in particular, are reviewed at FDA. The critical event was the unfolding of the hexachlorophene (HPC) saga. Some of you may not be aware of the incident which began this process. HPC, in addition to being an antimicrobial compound, is also a fairly good fungicide, and a proposal was made to use it as a fruit spray. Thus, toxicity studies were initiated to establish safe residue limits for food use.

EXPERIMENTAL STUDIES

The laboratory studies to establish the safety of HCP for use as a fungicide were initiated by Dr. Kimbrough and

co-workers in Atlanta (1, 2, 3). They observed toxic effects
of HCP in the rat after oral or dermal application of the
compound. A pronounced effect on the brain was produced in
rats fed 25 mg/kg/day, and toxicity was observed as early as
4 days after initiating treatment in adult rats. Increases
in wet weight of the brain occurred after 2 weeks of treatment with HCP and were greater after 4 weeks. Microscopic
examination of the rat brains exposed to this dose (equivalent to 500 ppm in the diet) showed vacuolated white matter
throughout the entire brain and spinal cord. With electron
microscopy, the vacuoles were observed to result from a
split in the interperiod line of the myelin sheath. Strands
of myelin were seen within the vacuoles. Weanling rats were
more susceptible and showed these effects after a single
100 mg/kg dose in 4 days. When 3% HCP was applied topically
daily for 30 days in detergent or propylene glycol, about
one-half the treated group of rats showed the same lesions
at 24 mg/kg/day.

Studies in the neonatal rhesus monkey were undertaken by
the Winthrop Laboratories (4). Newborn monkeys washed with
3% HCP for 90 days showed mean HCP plasma levels of 2.3 µg/
ml. Following sacrifice of the animals it was shown that
brain lesions identical to those described for the rat were
produced in monkeys receiving the topical application of
HCP (4).

Acute and chronic oral toxicity studies with HCP have
also been performed in animals. Single large doses produced
both neurologic and morphologic changes. Morphologic changes
have been associated with neurologic toxicity, brain and
spinal cord showing edematous changes and status spongiosus.
The white matter had expanded and showed large and small
vacuoles lined with myelin-staining strands of material.
The list of studies showing toxicity after the oral intravenous or topical administration of hexachlorophene in a
variety of animals is very long (2, 3).

CLINICAL DATA

The unfolding of the data on the clinical toxicity of HCP
demonstrates a very high degree of correlation with the experimental findings in animals. I believe Larson's study of
the absorption of HCP after burn treatment constitutes the
earliest description of clinical toxicity (5), and the neurologic symptoms occurring after the accidental oral ingestion
of HCP have been well described by Lockhart (6). Also, Dr.
Alvord's retrospective study in human infants who died of
other causes showed correlation of the specific status
spongiosus lesions with HCP-bathing of infants, especially

when the birth weight was low (7).

All of this information was a prelude to the final fit-
ting of the pieces together. The tragic French incident,
in which baby powder was inadvertently contaminated with
HCP, occurred in the midst of FDA's decision making process.
Discussions of both effectiveness and toxicity were being
pursued when data from these poisonings were made available
to FDA. With the advent of the French data, it could be
shown that the neurologic effects of HCP and the clinical
histopathology matched the animal data exactly. Also, by
this time it had become obvious that, whether HCP was given
orally or applied topically, the blood-level of HCP was an
important indicator of the toxic potential of the compound.

FDA CONCERNS

What was the "lesson from history?" It was really not
so surprising that high levels of HCP in the body could
produce neurologic disorder and morphologic changes. The
lesson for us was that *topically applied* hexachlorophene
could produce these effects. The pharmacologists and toxicologists were presented with an intriguing demonstration
of their hypotheses concerning topical applications and absorption of materials. Asked independently, prior to this
specific knowledge concerning HCP, these scientists would
have said, "abraded or denuded skin and occlusion will both
increase absorption"; indeed they did. Diapers, occlusive
covering, and a little almond oil, often used by French
mothers, may also have been an added filip to the presence
of hexachlorophene.

Two rather different but perhaps related areas concerning
hexachlorophene toxicity are troublesome and cause us a
twinge now and again. First, it is of concern that because
of the primary indicated use which remains for hexachlorophene, namely, as a surgical scrub and a handwashing product,
some individuals (up to 3%) may be repeatedly exposed to
topically applied HCP. Now, of course, we obtain data on
the blood concentration of chemicals after the exaggerated
use of hand-scrubbing products. With respect to HCP, in the
vast majority of cases the blood levels appear to be
plateaued after the 3-week test period of handwashing. However, as recorded in most such studies, a wide range of
blood values was found, and 2 or 3 subjects of a 30-person
test panel show levels significantly higher than the rest of
the group. The highest level reported from these tests is
0.87/µg/ml (ppm) (8). It is doubtful if the blood level of
HCP obtained after such scrubbing is harmful to the anatomically developed nervous system of an adult, but is this

also true if the person happens to be female and pregnant?
The toxicity from topically applied materials may go one
step further, that is, to the fetus. Based on the teratology
studies reported, it is assumed, if the reports are correct,
that HCP does cross the placental barrier. How does the
mother's blood level of HCP affect the developing neurologic
tissue of the fetus?

A second question of import has been raised over the
last 4 years, and keeps being raised to FDA, regarding the
reversibility of HCP-induced effects. The morphologic
changes in brain tissue associated with HCP appear to be reversible after withdrawal of the chemical. Dr. Alvord's
work in correlating lesions in newborns, especially in pre-
matures, with HCP bathing is well known (7), but this study
was done retrospectively from autopsy slides so that follow-
up was not possible. Dr. Pleuckhahn in Australia has at-
tempted to follow infants who have been exposed to HCP in
the hospital nursery, where HCP is still used to wash neo-
nates. A high correlation between HCP exposure, birth
weight, and the incidence of status spongiosus lesions has
been shown (9). He has assumed a high probability that in
cases where one of a set of twins dies in the hospital and
shows status spongiosus lesions that the surviving twin also
had them. Some of these children have been followed and
meet the rather general criteria of "functioning well."
Unfortunately, in dealing with this information one is
forced to base a final conclusion on a whole series of
cascading assumptions.

The conclusions being drawn from some of these observations are that the lesions may appear to be major but, since
the effect is probably reversible, there are probably no
apparent permanent sequelae. The difficulties inherent in
making this conclusion are that there has been a check for
only certain general effects. Perhaps the data which will
be forthcoming from the follow-up on the French infants who
were ill and had neurologic symptoms, but survived, will
provide additional objective data. Recent contact with
French officials of INCERN indicates that their follow-up is
very thorough and complete. Unfortunately one cannot observe the tissue repair or determine the biochemical activity of the affected tissue *in vivo*.

In addition a further specific lesion was reported in
rats in 1975 (10). Towfighi *et al.* found that 4-week old
rats given 900 ppm of HCP in the diet for varying times
showed disruption of the retinal disc membranes and of pho-
toreceptor outer segments and irreversible destruction of
their cell bodies. Early, probably reversible, changes
were vacuolation and vesiculotubular degeneration. Vacuolation in the disc was analogous to the lesions of the

white matter already mentioned. Irreversible changes occurred after 2 weeks or more.

Finally, I am sorry to report that, even as late as last week, suspected serious adverse reactions involving the misuse of products containing 3% HCP are still reported to FDA. Constant vigilance in the professional use of hexachlorophene-containing products is essential.

OTHER ANTIMICROBIALS

The FDA decision to remove hexachlorophene from many over-the-counter (OTC) products had an immediate effect on manufacturers producing these products. However, other effects are more lasting and pervasive. The OTC Antimicrobial 1 Panel, which recommended that action on HCP be taken immediately, also reviewed a number of other topical antimicrobials. The events I have described affected the remainder of the OTC review and effectively focused the Panel's attention on the absorption data available for other antimicrobial chemicals. In evaluating the data they were presented, many assumptions had to be made to establish a basis for determining safety factors from animal toxicity data when the same material is topically applied to humans.

The type of products being tested is critical. The Panel's review covers products ranging from antimicrobial soaps involving total-body-bathing daily to one-time applications of first-aid products. The possibility that absorption of a toxic ingredient from one of these topically applied materials may occur, with resultant systemic toxicity, was made obvious with HCP. Data submitted to the Panel showed that triclocarban, tribromsalan, and triclosan were absorbed following local application. Since many of these chemicals are excreted via the glucuronide pathway, there was concern about changes in excretory patterns if more than one chemical were applied at a time or if the glucuronide pathway were undeveloped, as it is in infants.

These and other factors have been considered and have been made a part of the extensive testing guidelines published as part of the OTC Antimicrobial I Panel's report (8). FDA has had at least one application for a new topical antimicrobial in which all of these tests have been considered and the appropriate ones performed. There are also several other proposed new antimicrobials which are being tested according to these Guidelines. Fortuitously, this antimicrobial is absorbed very slightly so that some of the tests in the Guidelines were not appropriate. In general these tests involve the following:

1. Tests on both the active ingredient and the formulated product.
2. Absorption studies in animals and humans with intact and abraded skin.
3. Blood-level determination for all tests, where appropriate, which means that a precise analytical procedure must be available.
4. The metabolic pathways must be examined and the effect on toxicity investigated as, for example, if impaired or undeveloped excretory pathways existed.

One other serious cutaneous toxicity problem that became more evident in the process of the OTC review is photosensitization by some salicylanilide-based antimicrobials, primarily tribomsalan or TBS. The details of this reaction, the human cases and the commentary on the Panel's report can be found both in the Panel's report and the Commissioner's final order removing it from the market (11). The problem and concern that this example presents to FDA is that of a very serious reaction with an extremely small incidence. It is frequently difficult or impossible to detect these reactions in clinical testing; if they are found it is often only a fortuitous occurrence.

SUMMARY

The examples reviewed demonstrate that predictive skin testing in both animals and humans is of value. Exaggeration of dose and means of application (frequency, occlusion and exposure to light) in these tests serve to provide FDA some confidence that release of products will not result in the marketing of potent or moderate sensitizers, photosensitizers, or irritants. In reference to Dr. Kligman's comments earlier, it is essential that FDA have available predictive tests. Perhaps the way to test for irritation, since the term predictive may not be applicable, is to do a comparative test with a range of compounds which includes known irritants, the test material, and a nonirritant.

Ultimately, when products do sensitize the rare individual, or even an established fraction of the population, risk/benefit ratio must be the final consideration. If animal and human testing results and, hopefully, incidence or prevalence data are available, the complex judgment of risk/benefit ratio is not only easier but is made on the results obtained from sound testing procedures.

Our awareness of topical absorption and the mechanisms which will increase it extend to chemical materials from unusual sources. For instance, residues from ethylene oxide

sterilization can be both toxic and irritating. Ethylene
chlorhydrin has been mentioned earlier as a toxic material.
FDA would now examine not only data on absorption of the
actual drug material but also information on the residual
chemicals from the sterilization process. Visualize for
example an impregnated bandage for serious burn treatment
which has been ethylene-oxide sterilized. Thus, the
history lesson of hexachlorophene has changed forever the
reviewing process and the toxicity data required for topically applied antimicrobial drug products.

REFERENCES

1. Gaines, T. B., and Kimbrough, R. D. (1971). The oral
    and dermal toxicity of hexachlorophene in rats. *Toxicol.*
    Appl. Pharmacol. *19*:375.
2. Kimbrough, R. D. (1971). Review of the toxicity of
    hexachlorophene. *Arch. Environ. Health* *23*:119.
3. Kimbrough, R. M. (1973). Review of recent evidence of
    toxic effects of hexachlorophene. *Pediatrics* *51*:391.
4. FDA (1971). Hexachlorophene and newborns. *FDA Drug*
    Bull. December.
5. Larson, D. L. (1968). Studies show hexachlorophene
    causes burn syndrome. *J. Amer. Hosp. Assoc.* *42*:63.
6. Lockhart, J. D. (1973). Hexachlorophene and the Food
    and Drug Administration. *J. Clin. Pharmacol.* *13*:445.
7. Shuman, R. M., Leech, R. W., and Alvord, E. C. (1974).
    Neurotoxicity of hexachlorophene in the human.
    Pediatrics, *54*:689.
8. OTC Antimicrobial I Panel Report (1974). *Fed. Regist.*
    39(179), September 13.
9. Plueckhahn, V. D. (1975). Central nervous system vacuo-
    lation in newly born infants, Nebourne, Australia, July
    1959 to June 1974. Draft copy presented to FDA, May
    1975. (In press.)
10. Towfighi, J., Gonatas, W. K., and McCree, L. (1975).
    Hexachlorophene retinopathy in rats. *Lab. Invest.* *32*:
    330.
11. *Fed. Regist.* (1972). *37*(188), September 27.

Toxicologic Perspectives
of Chemicals Commonly Applied to Skin

Howard I. Maibach

Department of Dermatology
University of California School of Medicine
San Francisco, California

Francis N. Marzulli

Toxicology Division
Food and Drug Administration
Washington, D.C.

In terms of frequency of application and contact area, cosmetics and skin-care products are among the products most commonly applied to human skin. They may be applied one or more times daily for a few days or a lifetime, and contact area may range from a few square centimeters (mascaras) to the entire body (soaps, bath oils, sunscreens). A knowledge of the safety of skin care preparations--individual ingredients and final formulations--is therefore important.

When skin-care products are used for a lifetime, it matters little whether they are called drug or cosmetic; the important issue is the need to resolve the question of their potential for cumulative topical and systemic effects.

The extent and sophistication of information sought by scientists of different disciplines are not the same. Cosmetic or pharmaceutical chemists who formulate and toxicologists and pharmacologists who evaluate do not have similar outlooks or philosophies. Neither do scientists in regulatory agencies, in industry, and in academia. The result is that product or ingredient safety is often a process of negotiation rather than of science when these scientists, operating from dissimilar vantage points, discuss this subject.

METHODS USED TO DETERMINE SAFETY

What are the information sources leading to decisions regarding the safety of commonly applied materials? Some of these materials have survived centuries of use because no adverse effects were documented. Most of them, however, are products of modern technology. As analytical methods and techniques for evaluation improve and our understanding of toxicologic potentials is increased, the newest chemicals are examined with increasing sophistication. Certain commonly applied materials of recent origin have survived because no undue hazard was detected in usage, and thus they have escaped careful scrutiny. With this appealing but hardly reliable approach, no overt hazard has been identified, but none has been sought. Recent examples of the toxic hazard missed with this approach are vinyl chloride and hexachlorophene (1).

The technique of epidemiology is difficult and expensive at best, and is especially forbidding when ubiquitous materials are involved. When a potential hazard is identified, it is sometimes possible to clarify its significance by "retrospective" predictive animal or human tests. In this manner, ethylene diamine and neomycin were found to be frequent sensitizers when proper diagnostic patch test methods were used on patients with eczema (2); in a normal population, these compounds remain rare sensitizers.

Much of the work on the chemicals under discussion was first performed in animals. Animal models are useful despite the fact that their relevance to man is often questioned. At first, animal tests provided only simple, routine toxicologic data such as acute toxicity (LD_{50}) and acute irritancy to skin or eye. Some models provide the background for similar studies in man, often using related techniques. The animal and human models detail the expected; they often do not foretell unexpected toxicity such as carcinogenesis, a compelling concern for chemical development in the future. One question which arose was "at what concentration do we test for irritancy in animals in order to extrapolate to man?" Testing in humans appears to resolve problems in human dermatotoxicology. This offers the advantage of working with the same species for which the chemical is ultimately intended, but does not permit one to determine serious acute or toxicologic effects. This important limitation can be overcome by the combined use of animal and human models.

In dermatotoxicology, useful human tests have been developed to assess skin irritation (3), skin sensitization (4), phototoxicity (5), photoallergy (6), and percutaneous penetration (7). Within the past decade, these tests have been improved and more accurately defined to increase their value.

Lastly, use experience--good and bad--has played a role in understanding toxicologic limitations of individual ingredients. For instance, information has been generated to provide guidelines for selecting the concentration of propylene glycol in various product categories that do not result in irritant dermatitis (8).

DERMATOTOXICOLOGY

Motivation for the development of new information on dermatotoxicology arises from different sources. Some responsible manufacturers of raw materials provide the results of several simple toxicologic tests about the chemicals they market. More often, the information released consists of one or two tests, i.e., an LD_{50} and acute eye or skin irritation. Occasionally, a more complete toxicologic profile, including extensive pharmacologic and toxicologic evaluations, is provided on both ingredient and specific examples of *final products*.

Antimicrobial agents used as preservatives have been among those substances studied in greater detail (9). A powerful stimulant was provided by the FDA Panel on Antimicrobial Agents which reviewed these substances following concern about the toxic implications of certain uses of hexachlorophene. It is unlikely, however, that the ideal of a complete toxicologic profile on each chemical and every combination proposed for contact with human skin will be achieved in the near future: regulatory activity, scientific, social, and economic aspects, and personal diligence are important factors in this equation. This interplay will determine how we approach the ideal.

Toxicologic Techniques

With the accumulation of data and the development of insight, pharmacologic and toxicologic techniques have been improved. Although new techniques tend to be used on new but not old chemicals, the concerned toxicologist is inclined to test both new and old chemicals by both the standard and improved techniques now available. A spirit of cooperation is needed among all involved parties in order to take advantage of technical advances as they occur.

Some members of industrial management may be inclined to question investigative methods they feel do not represent the real world. Some of these concerns are realistic, for some techniques are indeed difficult to extrapolate to human use. Other concerns may be simply due to a lack of understanding of the method or interpretation and a lack of other background information. The relevance of pharmacologic and toxicologic assays is discussed in detail in a recent text (10).

A better appreciation of dose, as employed in predictive assays versus use conditions, and greater insight are needed with regard to extrapolating from animals to man and from human assays to human use. An underemphasized approach entails the use of long-term follow-up on successes and failures of predictive techniques. Other experiences need to be recorded to improve our interpretation of data and techniques.

Systemic Absorption

Some scientists are convinced that the skin is an almost perfect barrier structure. This is in part true, for it is a remarkable membrane. Its most extraordinary property is its capacity for reducing (but not entirely preventing) water loss from the body. Transepidermal water loss in fact amounts to about 0.5 $mg/cm^2/hr$, a not insignificant amount (11). The skin's barrier properties for chemicals are quite different, however. Only in recent years have reliable quantitative data been obtained for a variety of chemicals (12) by *in vivo* techniques. The relative availability of radiolabeled chemicals has simplified analysis. For most chemicals examined with contemporary methods, at least 1% of the applied amount is absorbed; for many, significantly more is absorbed; and for some, as much as 50% is absorbed (12).

Table 1 relates the concentration of chemical applied to skin, the surface area, and the percentage absorbed, to determine the total amount that may be absorbed when a bath oil or sunscreen is applied to the entire body. To simplify the table, the percentage absorbed is stated for three points: 1, 10, and 50%. If a concentration of 1 $\mu g/cm^2$ is applied (which is in the range of a 0.06% concentration), only micrograms would be absorbed if 1% of the applied dose penetrated. If 10% was absorbed, this would raise the amount absorbed to the milligram range. For a chemical applied at 100 $\mu g/cm^2$ to the whole body, even a 1% absorption places the compound into a total in the milligram range. For compounds applied at 1 mg/cm^2, 10% absorption produces gram exposures. Using this data, repeated application of some commonly applied skin-care products is likely to result in considerable total systemic exposure.

Without reviewing the many steps involved in percutaneous penetration, it is more important to emphasize that most published human data on percutaneous penetration (*in vivo*)

TABLE 1

Factors that Affect the Relation between Amount Applied to Skin and Amount Absorbed

Concentration		Body surface		Amount applied		Percent absorbed		Total absorbed
1 µg/cm² (0.06%)	X	18,000 cm²	=	18 mg	X	1 10 50	=	180 µg 1.8 mg 9 mg
10 µg/cm² (0.6%)		18,000 cm²		180 mg		1 10 50		1.8 mg 18 mg 90 mg
100 µg/cm² (6.0%)		18,000 cm²		1.8 gm		1 10 50		18 mg 180 mg 900 mg
1000 µg/cm² (1 mg/cm²)		18,000 cm²		18 gm		1 10 50		180 mg 1.8 gm 9 gm

refs to the forearm (12). Some body sites allow considerably more absorption than the forearm: the ear, eyelid,
face, axilla, scalp, and cubital fossa are significantly more
permeable (13). The scrotum is virtually without barrier
properties. These and other factors must be considered when
discussing the potential for systemic toxicity with long-term
topical exposure.

Skin versus Other Routes of Expsoure in Animal Studies

Although oral or parenteral administration is simpler,
topical application provides a suitable route of exposure
for extrapolating animal toxicity to human use. Care must
be taken to avoid licking or other losses of applied material when unrestrained animals are used. Volatile materials
should be applied to animals in a fume hood to avoid inhalation. As the metabolic capacity of skin may be considerable
with some compounds, this possibility should be considered.
Furthermore, human and animal skin do not possess the same
enzyme systems and their metabolic capacities may differ
considerably.

COMMONLY APPLIED CHEMICALS

The Registration and Product Experience Branch, Division
of Cosmetics Technology of the Food and Drug Administration,
recently compiled a list of ingredients that appear in preparations marketed in the United States (Table 2); this information is based on voluntary submission of formulas by
cosmetics manufacturers. The table lists frequency of appearance of the ingredient without reference to the concentration in the formula and the frequency or contact area of
exposure. Despite these deficiencies, the list does provide
a sound basis for understanding the type of chemicals used
in cosmetics.
Table 3 lists the major categories that are pertinent to
the investigation of chemicals commonly applied to skin.
This is only an outline, and judgment must be used in determining relevance. For some items there is adequate background for interpretation, but for others the frame of reference is limited. The description of each category is not
definitive, but an attempt is made to demarcate some important factors relating to commonly applied materials.

Irritation Potential

This refers to epithelia of the skin, eyes, and mucous
membranes. The Draize test for skin irritation consists of

TABLE 2

Frequency of Cosmetic Ingredient Use as Voluntarily Reported by Cosmetic Manufacturers in the U. S.

Rank by Frequency	Frequency of use	Name of ingredient
1	4836	Water
2	2941	Methylparaben
3	2522	Propylparaben
4	1628	Mineral oil, light
5	1521	Propylene glycol
6	1482	Titanium dioxide
7	1449	Triethanolamine
8	1378	Cetyl alcohol
9	1286	Stearic acid
10	1181	Ferric oxide
11	1108	Talc
12	1099	Alcohol, 50 40
13	1045	Isopropyl myristate
14	970	Lanolin, anhydrous
15	923	FD & C yellow No. 5
16	815	Glycerin
17	760	Castor oil
18	680	FD & C blue No. 1
19	666	Carnauba wax
20	617	Beeswax, white
21	606	Propellant 12
22	579	Lanolin oil
23	535	Zinc stearate
24	534	Glyceryl monostearate
25	500	Alcohol, 50 39C
26	471	Ultramarine blue
27	453	Isopropyl alcohol
28	444	Candelilla wax
29	440	Mineral oil, heavy
30	433	Ozokerite
31	431	Oleyl Alcohol
32	429	Paraffin
33	414	Kaolin
34	413	Formaldehyde solution

TABLE 2 - *continued*

*Frequency of Cosmetic Ingredient Use as Voluntarily Reported
by Cosmetic Manufacturers in the U. S.*

Rank by Frequency	Frequency of use	Name of ingredient
35	400	D & C red No. 19
36	394	Magnesium aluminum silicate
37	388	Allantoin
38	370	D & C red No. 19-barium lake
39	366	Lanolin
40	358	Petrolatum
41	329	Sodium borate
42	303	Sodium lauryl sulfate
43	301	Sodium chloride
44	289	Lanolin alcohols
45	284	Microcrystalline wax
46	284	Citric acid
47	282	Magnesium carbonate
48	274	Polysorbate 20
49	270	Isopropyl palmitate
50	269	FD & C yellow No. 6
51	269	Polysorbate 60
52	266	Butylparaben
53	262	Zinc oxide
54	251	Propellant 114
55	249	Cetyl palmitate
56	245	Propellant 11
57	244	FD & C red No. 4
58	239	Stearyl alcohol
59	238	Ammonium hydroxide
60	225	Sorbic acid
61	223	Sorbitan sesquioleate
62	222	Menthol
63	217	Oleic acid
64	208	Beeswax, yellow
65	206	Ethyl alcohol
66	206	BHA
67	201	Propylene glycol monostearate

TABLE 3

Tests to be Performed on Suitable Animals and Then on Humans When Applicable, Appropriate, and Ethically Feasible[a]

---

1. Topical (skin). Determine:

a. Primary irritation potential following acute and subacute exposure. Special attention devoted to eyes, mucous membranes, and genitalia.

b. Allergic contact dermatitis potential following acute and subacute exposure.

c. Photosensitivity potential (phototoxic and photoallergenic). Tests to be conducted in appropriate age bracket in men and women and in sufficient numbers to determine safety.

d. Effect on wound healing.

e. Effect on skin pigmentation.

f. Effect on total skin flora to insure no detrimental over-growth of a particular bacterial or fungal species.

g. Substantivity or accumulation in or on the skin.

Note: The above tests should be performed using the chemical in pure form and in the final complete formulation to judge the effect of vehicle in the release of active ingredient(s).

2. Systemic. Determine:

a. The adequacy of or development of chemical analysis and/or bioassay techniques for the detection of the chemical and metabolites in biological tissues and secretions is essential.

b. Degree of absorption (blood level) through intact and abraded (damaged, diseased) skin and mucous membrane after acute and subchronic exposure. If the product is an aerosol, adequate inhalation studies should be conducted.

c. The target organ(s) for toxicity effects via oral, topical, and/or parenteral routes. Relate toxicity to blood levels of chemical agent. Determine the "no-effect" and "effect" level in the same species and same study.

d. The LD_{50}, highest dose killing no animals and lowest dose killing all the test animals by oral and topical route, if possible.

e. Tissue distribution, metabolic rates, metatolic fate, and rate and routes of excretion.

f. Teratogenic, mutagenic, carcinogenic, and reproductive effects.

TABLE 3 - *continued*

Tests to be Performed on Suitable Animals and Then on Humans When Applicable, Appropriate, and Ethically Feasible[a]

Note: The above tests should be performed using the chemical in pure form and in the final complete formulation to judge the effect of vehicle in the release of the active ingredient(s).

---

[a]From *Federal Register*, *39*(179), Sept. 13, 1974, 33135.

a single application of test material, under occlusion, to the clipped skin of rabbits (14). This technique was often used in the past to delineate the irritation potential of chemicals accidentally or intentionally brought in contact with skin. It has recently been modified and is sometimes recommended for use in conjunction with tests involving multiple application, depending on the type of chemical being investigated. Rather than relying on an arbitrary irritation index, as with the original Draize test, it may be more meaningful to compare a new or less known chemical with one for which there is considerable human experience. This provides a better reference standard in comparing new and old materials and can be done with individual ingredients or final formulations.

When operational definitions for irritancy were first developed, there was greater emphasis on relatively toxic chemicals such as those used in industry. At that time it was reasonable to define irritation as a dermatitis occurring after single nonimmunologic exposure. For most of the chemicals discussed here, a nonimmunologic dermatitis that might occur in only a few subjects after repeated application is of interest. This led to the development of cumulative irritancy testing (15, 16).

As noted, there is considerable information which permits the formulation chemist to make decisions on irritancy potential by utilizing the relative irritancy data on both single and multiple exposure.

Allergic Contact Dermatitis Potential

At one time, one might have hoped to perform these tests by *in vitro* techniques or by computer analysis. Presently, human test methods whose basic procedure was devised 20 years ago, with modifications, are used (17). By elevating the test concentration many times over use concentration it is possible to detect the sensitization potential of all but weak sensitizers (18). Adjuvant techniques employing guinea pig assays (19, 20) are used to detect weak sensitization potential, and the Draize-Landsteiner test (17) provides a measure of the test materials' capacity to detect strong sensitizers. The use of both tests provides a more complete assessment of sensitization potential. In addition, the use of adequate positive and negative controls provides an assessment of the technical ability of the investigator to perform the test correctly.

Phototoxicity Potential

Techniques for identifying phototoxic potential are now well developed (5, 21), and commonly applied materials are easily tested. Positive and negative controls are important. Bergapten and 8-methoxypsoralen are useful positive controls for substances activated by irradiation with light at 320-400 nm. Substances that fluoresce on irradiation are likely candidates for phototoxicity potential.

Photoallergic Potential

Photoallergy was poorly defined until the last decade. The major impetus for the development of new information in this area was provided by the episodes involving the halogenated salicylanilides (22). Most photosensitizers are also contact sensitizers. Most (but not all) of the photosensitizers have been identified in assays for contact sensitization. This area requires validating predictive models; the reader is referred to the Herman and Sams monograph for an extensive review (22).

Wound Healing

Many commonly used materials are placed on wounds or traumatized skin. Wound-healing models in animals and man are intended to ascertain whether any individual ingredient or final formulation would increase or decrease wound healing (23). Data of this kind are now available for some chemicals.

Skin Pigmentation

Occupational laukoderma was not described until World War II. Techniques for ascertaining this proclivity in both animals and humans are now available (24). Occupational leukoderma is easily misdiagnosed clinically as vitiligo. Only when assays are done for depigmentation potential of

commonly applied chemicals can we separate endogenous (vitiligo) from exogenous (environmental chemicals) depigmentation.

Skin Flora

Techniques for quantitating skin bacteria have improved.
Many common chemicals such as propylene glycol are potent
antimicrobial agents. Some chemicals not ordinarily considered to be antimicrobial (e.g., scopolamine) do in fact
have such properties when examined by appropriate *in vitro*
assay. How does this affect the cutaneous microbial ecology
of man in health and disease? This is an area in which further work should be done. When is it appropriate to develop
information on the effect of a given chemical on the skin
flora? For established antimicrobials, the decision is easy,
but for other chemicals it may be more difficult. Recently,
an attempt was made to define this effect for one commonly
used antimicrobial agent (25).

Substantivity

Percutaneous pharmacokinetics of a chemical cannot be
properly interpreted without knowledge of its substantivity
(retention on skin). Methods have been developed for quanti-
tation (7). It is hoped that such information will be
available for chemicals commonly used on human skin.

Systemic Exposure

Percutaneous penetration is a complex matter. It consists of at least ten individual steps, each of which is
important (7). For instance, a compound may be minimally
absorbed and yet offer a significant toxic potential if it
is incompletely or slowly excreted; heavy metals such as
lead and mercury are examples (26). Hexachlorophene is a
minimal skin penetrant of normal adult skin. Its adverse
systemic effects occur because of its substantivity (which
accounts for prolonged skin penetration) and its high inherent toxicity. Many assays to characterize systemic toxic
potential are rapid and efficient such as the acute LD_{50};
others are slow, cumbersome, and expensive such as those
necessary to determine carcinogenicity and reproductive
effects.

SPECIFICS: PROPYLENE GLYCOL

Propylene glycol is the third most commonly used

compound listed in Table 2. It has probably been subjected
to more intensive study than most others listed among the
top ten. Nevertheless, a critical evaluation of available
information about this compound discloses some weaknesses
and a lack of completeness.

Propylene glycol (organic alcohol, $C_3H_8O_2$;1,2-propanediol)
is a clear, colorless, hygroscopic, viscous liquid that is
miscible with water, acetone, alcohol, and chloroform and is
soluble in ether. It is used as a solvent, humectant, con-
stituent of hydrophilic ointment USP, and aerosol antiseptic
(27, 28). Cosmetic specifications have been established by
the Cosmetic, Toiletry, Fragrance Association, Inc. (29).
It can be procured from Union Carbide Co. (30).

Toxic Potential

This compound has had a relatively long and extensive
history of use, study, and toxicologic evaluation. Its
toxicity is said to be similar to that of glycerin, which
is thought to be practically nontoxic (31). A summary of
acute LD_{50}'s by various routes in animal species (Table 4)
reveals that propylene glycol has a low inherent toxicity
(32).

Long-term (2 year) oral toxicity studies in rats (33)
showed that there were no significant toxic effects or
carcinogenic potential after ingestion of up to 5% propylene
glycol in the diet. This is equivalent to 2.5 g/kg/day or
1.8 g/day in a 70 kg man. Similar data (daily exposures)
are not available for *topical* exposure.

In 1974, propylene glycol was evaluated for acceptable
daily intake by the joint FAO/WHO Expert Committee on Food
Additives (34). In this evaluation, it was concluded that
up to 25 mg/kg would be an acceptable daily intake for man.
This was based mainly on animal toxicity data. In this report, the biochemistry, acute toxicity, short- and long-term
toxicity studies in animals, and exploratory work in man
were reviewed.

The carcinogenic and toxicologic potential of propylene
glycol by repeated (twice weekly) skin application to mice
over their life-span disclosed no adverse effects on skin
or other organs (35).

Propylene glycol was found to be relatively nonirritating
to man and rabbits when used as such or when diluted (10% and
50% in water) (36). Tests consisted of single and multiple
(21 day) exposures using uncovered and covered skin.

In primary irritation studies on rabbits, piglets, and
man, undiluted propylene glycol was reported to produce only
minimal skin reactions (37). Effects on the skin were said
to be similar in these species and man. In the mouse,

TABLE 4

LD$_{50}$ of 1,2-Propanediol

Species	Route	LD$_{50}$[a]	Reference
Rat	po	30.0(5) (40%)[b]	Weatherby and Haag (1938)
		21.0(10)	Laug *et al.* (1939)
		28.0(5)	Thomas *et al.* (1949)
		28.8(?)	Merck Index (1969)
	im	15.0(5) (60%)	Braun and Cartland (1936)
		13.0(10) (40%)	Seidenfeld and Hanzlik (1932)
		20.0(5)	Thomas *et al.* (1949)
		14.0(5) (60%)	Weatherby and Haag (1938)
	sc	22.0(5) (60%)	Braun and Cartland (1936)
		25.0(5) (80%)	Weatherby and Haag (1938)
		28.0(5)	Thomas *et al.* (1949)
	iv	7.0(5) (80%)	Weatherby and Haag (1938)
		15.0(10) (40%)	Seidenfeld and Hanzlik (1932)
	ip	13.0(5)	Thomas *et al.* (1949)
Mouse	po	23.9(20)	Laug *et al.* (1939)
	iv	4.8(?)	Lehmann and Flury (1943)
	ip	10.9(10)	Davis and Jenner (1959)
Rabbit	po	18.0(9) (33%)	Braun and Cartland (1936)
		19.0(7) (86%)	Braun and Cartland (1936)
	im	6.0(3) (33%)	Seidenfeld and Hanzlik (1932)
	iv	5.0(3) (66%)	Seidenfeld and Hanzlik (1932)
		7.0(5) (80%)	Weatherby and Haag (1938)
Guinea pig	po	18.9(10)	Laug *et al.* (1939)
Dog	po	20.0(?)	Laug *et al.* (1939)

[a]Expressed as mg per kg body weight. Number of animals in dose group is given in parentheses.
[b]Percent selected to represent LD$_{50}$.

guinea pig, miniature pig, dog, and baboon effects were even less prominent than those observed in man.

Some investigators have reported that propylene glycol may produce skin sensitization in man, but other investigators were unable to produce skin sensitization in experimental studies in man using 293 subjects (18). The published assays of allergic contact dermatitis sensitization potential leave some questions unanswered as to whether sensitization does or does not exist. The recent publication of Hannuksela should be consulted for further details (38).

It may be concluded that propylene glycol does not appear to possess overt toxicologic or other adverse properties when evaluated as a cosmetic ingredient. Although a complete evaluation would require that it be tested in combination with other ingredients, there is no reason to believe that this compound would prove to be unsafe for use in cosmetics under favorable conditions of use, based on its known chemical, physical, and toxicologic properties.

CONCLUSIONS

Unfortunately, reasonable information on phototoxic potential, photoallergic potential, effects on wound healing, effects on skin pigmentation, alteration of skin flora, substantivity, amount of percutaneous penetration in man, excretion in man, tissue distribution, teratology, mutagenicity, and reproductive effects are not fully documented. Should this be cause for concern? That depends upon your viewpoint. No matter what the viewpoint--that of the raw material supplier, the user, or the scientist in regulatory affairs--it would be ideal and perhaps not too difficult to close the gaps. Only when this information is available will we know if important hazards in a chemical's clinical use are being missed.

There are extensive pharmacologic and toxicologic data on some commonly applied chemicals. Some scientists undoubtedly believe this is adequate. Others conclude that it is adequate in terms of documented hazard, but inadequate in terms of defining each potential hazard. Efficient ways of gaining the additional information should be sought and a modus operandi for reexamining the older chemicals using better assay methods must be developed.

More effective ways of determining the hazards to man, especially for those chemicals most commonly applied, must be more clearly defined.

REFERENCES

1. Marzulli, F. N., and Maibach, H. (1975). Relevance of animal models: The hexachlorophene story. In *Animal Models in Dermatology*, ed. H. Maibach, pp. 156-167. New York, Churchill Livingstone.
2. Bandmann, H. J., Calnan, C. D., Cronin, E., *et al.* (1971). Dermatitis from applied medicaments. *Arch. Dermatol. 106*:335.
3. Steinberg, W., Akers, W., Weeks, M., McCreech, A., and Maibach, H. (1975). A comparison of test techniques based on rabbit and human skin responses to irritants with recommendations regarding the evaluation of mildly or moderately irritating compounds. In *Animal Models in Dermatology*, ed. H. Maibach, pp. 1-11. New York, Churchill Livingstone.
4. Buehler, E., and Griffith, J. (1975). Experimental skin sensitization in the guinea pig and man. In *Animal Models in Dermatology*, ed. H. Maibach, pp. 56-66. New York, Churchill Livingstone.
5. Marzulli, F., and Maibach, H. (1975). Phototoxicity (photoirritation) from topical agents. In *Animal Models in Dermatology*, ed. H. Maibach, pp. 84-89. New York, Churchill Livingstone.
6. Harber, L., and Shalita, A. (1975). The guinea pig as an effective model for the demonstration of immunologically mediated contact photosensitivity. In *Animal Models in Dermatology*, ed. H. Maibach, pp. 98-102. New York, Churchill Livingstone.
7. Maibach, H., Feldmann, R., and Marzulli, P. (1977). Ten steps in percutaneous penetration. In *Advances in Modern Toxicology*, ed. F. Marzulli and H. Maibach. Washington, D. C., Hemisphere (in press).
8. Maibach, H. (1976). (unpublished).
9. Dept. of HEW, FDA, O-T-C Topical Antimicrobial Products and Drug and Cosmetic Products. *Fed. Regist. 39*(179), Part II, Sept. 13, 1974.
10. Maibach, H. (1975) (ed.) *Animal Models in Dermatology: Relevance to Human Dermatopharmacology and Dermatotoxicology*. New York, Churchill Livingstone.
11. Blank, I. H. (1953). Further observations on factors which influence the water content of the stratum curneum. *J. Invest. Dermatol. 21*:259.
12. Feldmann, R., and Maibach, H. (1970). Absorption of some organic compounds through the skin in man. *J. Invest. Dermatol. 54*:399.
13. Maibach, H., Feldmann, R., Milby, R., and Serat, W. (1971). Regional variation in percutaneous penetration in man. *Arch. Environ. Health 23*:208.

14. Draize, J., Woodard, G., and Calbery, H. (1944). Methods for the study of irritation and toxicity of substances applied topically to the skin and mucous membranes. *J. Pharmacol. Exp. Ther.* *82*:337.

15. Phillips, L., Steinberg, M., Maibach, H., and Akers, W. (1972). A comparison of rabbit and human skin responses to certain irritants. *Toxicol. Appl., Pharmacol.* *21*:369.

16. Marzulli, F., and Maibach, H. (1975). The rabbit as a model for evaluating skin irritants: A comparison of results obtained on animals and man using repeated skin exposures. *Food and Cosmet. Toxicol.* *13*:533.

17. Draize, J. H., (1959). Dermal toxicity. In *Appraisal of the Safety of Chemicals in Foods, Drugs and Cosmetics*. Austin, Texas, Association of Food and Drug Officials of the United States.

18. Marzulli, F., and Maibach, H. (1974). Use of graded concentrations in skin sensitizers: Experimental contact sensitization in man. *Food and Cosmet. Toxicol.* *12*:219.

19. Magnusson, B., and Kligman, A. (1970). *Allergic Contact Dermatitis in the Guinea Pig*. Springfield, Ill., Thomas.

20. Maguire, H. C., Jr. (1973). The bioassay of contact allergens in the guinea pig. *Soc. Cosmet. Chem.* *24*: 151.

21. Maibach, H., and Marzulli, F. (1977). Phototoxicity. In *Advances in Modern Toxicology*, ed. F. Marzulli and H. Maibach, Washington, D. C., Hemisphere (in press).

22. Herman, P., and Sams, W. M. (1972). *Soap Photodermatitis*. Springfield, Ill., Thomas.

23. Maibach, H., and Rovee, D. (1972) (eds.). *Epidermal Wound Healing*. Chicago, Year Book Publishers.

24. Gellin, G. (1975). Prediction of human depigmenting chemicals with the guinea pig. In *Animal Models in Dermatology*, ed. H. Maibach, pp. 267-271. New York, Churchill, Livingstone.

25. Aly, R., and Maibach, H. (1976). Effects of antimicrobial soap containing chlorhexidene on the microbial flora of skin. *Appl. Environ. Microbiol.* *31*:931.

26. Marzulli, F., and Brown, D. W. C. (1972). Potential Systemic hazards of topically applied mercurials. *J. Soc. Cosmet. Chem.* *23*:875.

27. Gleason, M. N., Gosselin, R., Hodge, H., and Smith, R. (1969). *Clinical Toxicology of Commercial Products*, 3rd Ed. Baltimore, Md., The Williams & Wilkins Co.

28. *Remington's Pharmaceutical Sciences*, 15th Ed., (1975). Easton, Pa., Mack Publishing Co.

29. *The Merck Index*, 8th Ed. (1968), ed. Paul G. Stecher. Rahway, N.J., Merck and Co., Inc.

30. Cosmetic, Toiletry and Fragrance Assoc., Inc., 1133 Fifteenth St., N.W., Wash., D.C. 20008

31. Union Carbide Corp. - Chemicals Div., 270 Park Ave., New York, N.Y. 10017.

32. Ruddick, J. A. (1972). Toxicology, metabolism, and biochemistry of 1,2-propanediol. *Toxicol. Appl. Pharmacol. 21*:102.

33. Gaunt, I. F., Carpanini, F. M., Grasso, P., and Lansdown, A. B. G. (1972). Long-term toxicity of propylene glycol in rats. *Food Cosmet. Toxicol. 10*:151.

34. World Health Organization (1974). Toxicological evaluation of some food additives including anticaking agents, antimicrobials, antioxidants, emulsifiers and thickening agents. 520, xix p. *ITS* WHO Food Additives Series, No. 5, p. 491. Also issued as FAO Nutrition Meetings Report Series, No. 53A.

35. Stenbach, F., and Shubik, P. (1974). Lack of toxicity and carcinogenicity of some commonly used cutaneous agents. *Toxicol. Appl., Pharmacol. 30*:7.

36. Phillips, L., Steinberg, M., Maibach, H., and Akers, W. (1972). A comparison of rabbit and human skin responses to certain irritants. *Toxicol. Appl. Pharmacol. 21*:369.

37. Davies, R. E., Harper, K., and Kynoch, S. R. (1972). Inter-species variation in dermal reactivity. *J. Soc. Cosmet. Chem. 23*:371.

38. Hannuksela, M., Pirila, V., and Salmo, O. (1975). Skin reactions to propylene glycol. *Contact Dermatitis 1*:112.

Cosmetic Legislation:
A Congressional Viewpoint

Senator Thomas F. Eagleton

Washington, D.C.

There has been a growing public awareness and concern over the last decade about the environmental hazards posed by substances that are potentially toxic, carcinogenic, mutagenic, or teratogenic. Every day we are exposed to so many chemicals and chemical compounds that even if only a small fraction of them should prove to be harmful they represent a very substantial threat to public health.

The publicized hazards associated with chemicals like vinyl chloride, BCME (bis[chloromethyl]ether), asbestos, PCBs (polychlorinated biphenyls), DES (diethylstilbestrol), and all of the others have dramatically illustrated how important it is that some system be established to give an early warning with respect to new chemical substances and to empower the appropriate authorities to gather test data and to take necessary regulatory action with respect to existing chemicals.

Taking carcinogenic substances as one example, the Secretary of Health, Education, and Welfare, in his department's Forward Plan for Health, reported estimates that 80 to 90% of all cancer is environmentally induced. If smoking and other personal factors are excluded, the largest portion of the remaining cancer is produced as a result of exposure to toxic substances in the work place, with a substantial portion occurring as a result of occupational exposures.

For all of these reasons, Congress and the Executive

Branch have taken a number of actions over the past decade
with respect to the discovery and regulation of harmful and
potentially harmful substances.

One of the most significant governmental actions in my
judgment, but also one of the least noted, was the establishment of the National Institute of Environmental Health Sciences (NIEHS) about 9 years ago. This institute, located in
the Research Triangle of North Carolina, is charged with conducting research that will enable scientists to identify
toxic agents in advance, rather than noting their effects on
the consumers who are too often used as involuntary human
guinea pigs.

The Institute has focused much of its attention on development of new screening tests that will greatly abbreviate
the time, effort, and expense required by most current test
processes. As many of you are aware, a complete toxicological test today may take 2 or 3 years and require considerable
resources of test animals and trained manpower. With up to
2,000,000 substances already in distribution...with 13,000
substances listed in the toxic substances list of the
National Institute of Occupational Safety and Health...and
with 600 to 1,000 new substances entering the market every
year...the time and expense required for testing becomes
of extraordinary significance.

One of the research activities now being undertaken by
NIEHS that has greatly impressed me is the effort to validate
the test developed by Dr. Bruce Ames, in which bacteria,
rather than animals, are used for testing. As most of you
are probably aware, Dr. Ames used *Salmonella* bacteria to test
the mutagenic effects--and thus, inferentially, the carcinogenic effects--of questioned substances. Using the Ames
Test, substances can be screened in a matter of 2 days at a
cost ranging from $600 to $1,500. As a member of the Senate
Appropriations Subcommittee dealing with health matters, I
intend to do all I can to see that the work of the Environmental Health Sciences Institute is given adequate support.

The question of developing efficient and cheap tests has
considerable bearing on the recurring argument over premarket
testing and premarket clearance of consumer products. As
might be expected, industry maintains that statutory requirements that products be tested and the tests submitted to a
federal agency for clearance before marketing results in
such costs and is so time-consuming that the affected industry is severely penalized. Consumer advocates, on the other
hand, point to the clear and present danger to which the public has been exposed over the years by such chemicals as
vinyl chloride and PCBs to demonstrate that premarket testing and clearance are absolutely essential in any regulatory
scheme.

Two pending items of legislation reflect the differing congressional approaches that have been taken to this issue. The two are the toxic substances bill and the cosmetic safety bill. The toxic substances legislation has passed the Senate and is now being considered by the House. The cosmetic safety bill, which I authored, has been ordered reported by the Senate Labor and Public Welfare Committee and will be taken up by the full Senate in the next few weeks.

By way of background, statutory requirements respecting premarket clearance are currently limited primarily to pesticides, drugs, and food additives. Industry cites the experience in these areas to illustrate the long delays that are necessarily occasioned by making government agencies responsible for clearing products prior to marketing.

This debate came to a head in the hearings conducted over the past several years on the cosmetic safety bill. As originally drafted, the bill provided that cosmetics must be cleared by the FDA in the same way as new drug applications are processed. Both industry and the FDA contended that such an elaborate screening mechanism was not necessary in the case of cosmetics, arguing that the threat to health they present is not sufficiently grave to require premarket clearance. Moreover, FDA maintained that such additional burdens would impair its ability to fulfill its major responsibilities in the area of food and drugs. Cosmetic manufacturers pointed out that the fashion industry is a seasonal one that demands a rapid entry into the market place if a product is to be competitive.

Consumer representatives maintain, however, that cosmetics are responsible for many thousands of injuries every year, estimated by the Consumer Product Safety Commission to amount to 60,000 a year. This threat, say the consumerists, justifies the imposition of strict standards for testing and clearance before any cosmetic can be marketed.

The bill approved by the committee adopts neither of these positions. It requires that cosmetic products be tested before they are marketed. However, test results need not be submitted to the FDA for premarket clearance. Rather, the FDA is authorized to request such data from manufacturers whenever it perceives that some health threat may exist. Manufacturers are obliged to retain test data and such other information as may be necessary to substantiate the safety of their products. Any consumer complaints they receive must be forwarded to the FDA.

As I envision operations under this bill, the FDA, acting on the basis of consumer complaints or other information, could order all manufacturers using a particular questioned substance in their products to submit test data. Since the bill requires manufacturers to register their names, ad-

dresses, and product formulas with the FDA, the identification and notification of affected manufacturers should be
relatively simple. If the FDA finds there is inadequate data
to substantiate the safety of the product, it may either ban
it from the market place or order additional testing, depending on the degree of public health hazard involved.

Thus, the cosmetic safety bill imposes on manufacturers
the legal obligation of substantiating the safety of their
products through premarket testing, but does not require
them to submit safety data for clearance prior to marketing.

The toxic substances bill takes a different tack. Under
the Senate-passed bill, manufacturers of new chemical substances must notify the Environmental Protection Agency (EPA)
90 days before such substances are to be manufactured. If
required by the EPA, they must also submit test data. I
suspect that, in most cases, the Administrator of EPA will
feel that he is obliged either to approve or to disapprove
the proposed new substances. He will therefore require the
submission of test data and the process will be one of premarket clearance. The FDA Administrator is further authorized to require manufacturers to test or have tested those
chemical substances which he determines may present an unreasonable risk of injury to health or the environment or
those for which significant human or environmental exposure
takes place or will take place. This provision is applicable both to new and existing chemical substances.

These bills represent different approaches to the central
issue of premarket testing and clearance based upon a congressional assessment of the gravity of the risk to public
health involved. I think that a sensible balance was struck
in each case. Both bills create a regulatory apparatus
within which the appropriate federal agencies are authorized
to take the steps necessary to protect the public health
without adding unduly to the cost of production--costs which
ultimately have to be paid by the consumer, of course.

Whether or not Congress is going to be able to continue
making such reasoned judgments, relating stringency of regulation to the degree of risk involved, remains to be seen.
There are strong countervailing forces in each direction.

Some consumer interests argue with great passion and conviction that industry can never be trusted to participate in
the regulatory process. Pointing to recent disclosures of
the Senate Health Subcommittee regarding drug tests, they
maintain that federal agencies should not even rely on data
from tests conducted or sponsored by industry, but that
testing by independent sources should be required.

Some elements in industry argue with equal passion and
conviction that government is undermining free enterprise
system by overregulation in pursuit of an impossible goal--

the risk-free society.

There are, of course, more moderate voices in each camp. But the net effect is that Congress is being pressured to choose one course or the other--either to require the testing and clearance of the enormous range and variety of substances which affect the consumer and his environment, or else to leave it to industry to assure the safety of its products, with the consumer's major recourse being the right of private legal action after damages have been suffered.

I don't believe either of these is an acceptable policy for Congress to adopt. We should continue to be in a position to view each regulatory proposal on its own merits. The degree and kind of regulation authorized by Congress ought to be reasonably related to the degree and kind of risk to the public that is involved.

I urge each of you--whether you represent the consumer movement, or private industry, or whether you exemplify the spirit of free inquiry which is fundamental to scientific investigation--that you work with us in providing the support and, most importantly, the information essential to the proper exercise of congressional responsibilities in this area.

INDEX